Acumoxa Therapy

A Reference and Study Guide

Acumoxa Therapy

A Reference and Study Guide

Paul Zmiewski and Richard Feit

"The method of deliverance:

the miraculous needle!"

— Dou Jie, *Ode to Elucidate Mysteries*

Paradigm Publications   *Brookline, Massachusetts*

1989

ISBN 0-912111-22-4

Library of Congress Cataloging in Publication Data

Zmiewski, Paul.
   Acumoxa therapy : comprehensive reference & study guide / Paul
Zmiewski.
         p.   cm
   Bibliography: p.
         Includes index.
         ISBN 0-912111-22-4 : $19.95
         1. Moxa.   I. Title.
         RM306.Z55 1989
         615.8'92--dc19   89-2989

Paradigm Publications

Publisher: Robert Felt
Editor: Richard Feit
Art and Design: Laura Shaw

Typesetting Software
by
Textware International, Cambridge, Massachusetts

Contents

Part IV   Pathology: Causes and Patterns of Disease

Part V   Diagnosis

Acknowledgements

The contributions and suggestions of many good people have made this present work possible. We especially wish to thank Peter Valaskatgis for his careful review and revision of the TCM point formulae found in Chapter 18; Susan Goldbaum for her review of the clean needle technique information; and Michael Hussin for his review of the five-phase system of qi transfer.

We would also thank Nigel Wiseman and Paul Unschuld, to whose works we constantly turn for clarification, inspiration and the deepening of our own understanding of Chinese Medicine.

It is our hope this new work will provide a favorable contribution to the ever-improving body of literature on acupuncture and Oriental medicine. We welcome your comments, suggestions, corrections, and criticisms, and promise to faithfully review them and include them, when appropriate, in future editions.

P.Z.
R.F.

Brookline, Massachusetts
March, 1989

Introduction

As universal in scope and sparkling with insights as are the fundamental principles of Oriental medicine, there is, lurking in the background of every Oriental medical student's experience, a sobering reality. The bewildering array of detail that gives form to these principles must, at some point, be memorized, organized, and applied. Sooner or later, in the classroom, for licensure, or in the clinic, the tests will begin to appear.

Students of Oriental medicine share this woe with students of all other disciplines. However, unlike other students, Western students of Oriental medicine have not had the advantage of review texts and study guides to help them in their times of trial. For many, even a good compilation would have been a book to cherish.

Though lamentable, this situation has been understandable. The Oriental medical profession in the West hadn't settled down long enough for an effective compilation to be undertaken, and publishers have been largely preoccupied with the steady stream of *new* works and translations.

Thus, the student, the new applicant for licensure, and the beginner in practice have been left without a dependable, single source for review and directed self study. It is to them that we have dedicated this effort.

A Few Words About Organization

You have in your hand a general review of acumoxa theory, presented in table format, and organized like a system of directories, files and notecards.

Being a general review, *Acumoxa Therapy* presents a compilation of the basic, fundamental theories and techniques found in most modern texts on Chinese medicine, both in Chinese and in English, and in most schools in China and the West. It is intended to accompany formal instruction, and to provide a source for ongoing review after formal instruction has been completed. It does not pretend to present the entirety of Chinese acumoxa theory, nor the many different schools of thought that comprise the practice of acupuncture today, or that have existed over the centuries. Indeed, such a task can only be accomplished through the formal study of a wide variety of texts with a variety of teachers and preceptors (the Bibliography offers a guide for such ongoing and in-depth study). Nor does this volume cover point and channel anatomy (point location and channel trajectories), topics that are complete studies in themselves, and that must be presented in highly specific detail (again, see the Bibliography for appropriate texts).

Seven large sections (Parts I-VII) comprise the directories of the file system: Basic Theory; Channels; Points; Pathology; Diagnosis; Strategies for Point Selection; and Clinical Practice.

Each Part begins with its own summarized table of contents listing the chapters to be found within it and the tables (here indicated by a •) found within those chapters. Tables have been used throughout the book as the primary means for presentation of the information. Occasionally, where some context is helpful or when a point needs to be underscored, tables are accompanied by short introductory or clarifying remarks.

Two kinds of tables are used — *standard tables* and *overview tables*. Standard tables are the notecards in the filing system, and contain the bulk of the detailed information presented in the text. Overview tables are less frequently encountered, and are somewhat more specialized in their intent.

Overview tables are found at the head of each part and at the beginning of some chapters, and may be distinguished by their double-line border. They present a highly distilled, and therefore generalized, version of the information about to be presented. The table on pages 38 and 39, "17 Important Point Types and Categories," is an example of an overview table. Notice that the left-most column of this table is also a list of the standard tables that immediately follow. This practice holds true for most other overview tables throughout the text.

Overview tables have two purposes: they allow you to *preview* the information about to be presented (in effect, they tell you what you are about to study); and, when study is complete, they provide a focused *review* of the information studied. Study the overview tables first to define the essential material of the section. Return to the overview tables to test recall and to re-establish the context within which the detailed information may be understood.

In addition to appearing within the body of the text, all overview tables are presented as a group in the first of the appendices. Look to this appendix as a further aid to review: it is a highly condensed tour through the basic tenets of acumoxa therapy.

English and Chinese References

English sources referenced to compile this manual include such standards as *Essentials of Chinese Acupuncture*, the newer *Chinese Acupuncture and Moxibustion*, *Acupuncture, a Comprehensive Text*, *Fundamentals of Chinese Medicine*, *Fundamentals of Chinese Acupuncture*, and *Nan-Ching: Classic of Difficult Issues*. Wherever appropriate, references will be made to the pages in these books where the reader can find more information on the subject at hand. Other sources that have been consulted more for comparison are listed in the bibliography only. Chinese sources used are referenced more casually; a complete list may be found in the bibliography. See the key at the end of this introduction for abbreviations used when English texts have been referenced.

A Short Note on Terminology

A great deal of fulminant downpour has precipitated lately over the issue of Chinese medical terminology in English, particularly since the publication of *Fundamentals of Chinese Medicine*. That work took a purposefully radical approach, one that was toned down to some extent in the authors' next book, *Fundamentals of Chinese Acupuncture*. But the translators' guiding principle remained the same: **term distinctions made in Chinese must be preserved in English**. It is not really important what particular word choices a translator makes; what is really important is that choices are indeed made, and that they are consistent within the system created. To date, only two translators, Nigel Wiseman and Paul Unschuld, have attempted this level of linguistic and etymological veracity in their works.

However, while linguistic precision may reflect the sense-meaning of the original term in the source language, it does not necessarily aid in clarifying the sense of the term in its clinical context. While "efflux desertion" is etymologically the most accurate and precise rendering of the Chinese *hua tuo*, it does not necessarily give the student any hint that this term refers to various forms of critical fluid loss, the most common being the fulminant diarrhea associated with dysentery or cholera. Consequently, other translators have emphasized a clinical, rather than a scholastic, orientation. While their word choices may not be as etymologically precise as Wiseman's or Unschuld's, they often reflect the clinical language encountered in daily medical practice with modern Chinese practitioners. Medical practitioners, whether Chinese or Western, have always used a more casual jargon among themselves to refer to clinical entities described more precisely in their medical textbooks. It should be borne in mind, however, that these "linguistic shortcuts" are taken by experienced practitioners already familiar with the subtleties of Chinese differential diagnosis, and may prove a pitfall for the still inexperienced student, preventing him or her from truly grasping the underlying concepts associated with any particular term.

What must be avoided, at all costs, is a false presentation of Chinese medical theory, i.e., a presentation based on the particular conceptual bias of the translator. If one chooses to translate only those concepts that he or she feels conceptually valid, disregarding the rest, the non-Chinese speaking student will be presented with only a partial picture of Chinese medicine, one that is quite different than that presented to his Chinese-speaking counterpart — one that is bound to be inconsistent and incoherent. While it is undoubtedly true that there is considerable detritus in the vast body of Chinese medical theory, it is not the province of the translator to determine what is valid and what is not.

With this in mind, we have attempted here to reconcile certain fundamental terminologic discrepancies found in the various texts referenced. We have our own prejudices, to be sure. They will be evident in the text and do not merit discussion here. Wherever a disputed term is used, at least at its first occurrence, alternative terms are also given. For the best discussion of the varied approaches to Chinese medical term translation, and the problems encountered, the reader is referred to the collection of papers presented at the First International Symposium on Chinese Medical Literature held at the University of Munich in 1986, entitled *Approaches to Traditional Chinese Medical Literature* (Dordrecht: Kluwer Academic Publishers, 1988), edited by Paul Unschuld.

Key to Abbreviations and Notations	
ACT	*Acupuncture, a Comprehensive Text* (Bensky, O'Connor)
CAM	*Chinese Acupuncture and Moxibustion* (Beijing College of T.C.M.)
TFCM	*Theoretical Foundations of Chinese Medicine (Porkert)*
†	Indicates moxa application
•	In tables of contents, indicates a standard table

Part I

Basic
Theory

The theoretical foundations of modern Chinese acumoxa therapy are based on four fundamental concepts:

(1) The concept of **yin and yang**;

(2) The differentiation of **qi, blood, body fluids,** and **essence** as the substantial components of body function;

(3) The **organs**, considered in paired yin-yang, interior-exterior groups, each with its own specialized role in maintaining life functions;

(4) The **five phases** of organ/system interaction, which explain functional interrelationships within the living organism.

1 Yin and Yang

Yin-Yang theory maintains that all things are essentially composed of two opposing, yet complementary, aspects, and that all phenomena naturally group themselves into complementary pairs of opposites. In Chinese medicine, this theory extends to physiology, anatomy, pathology, pharmaceutics, diagnosis, and treatment.

1.1 Yin-Yang relationships

It is important at the outset to have a general overview of yin-yang theory as it relates to general phenomena, physiological structures (body regions, tissues and organs), physiological activities, and general illness patterns. Yin-yang categorizations of pulses are also introduced here: more specific diagnostic indicators of yin-yang patterns will be presented in **Part IV, Pathology**.

General Yin-Yang Relationships	
Phenomena	Space, Time, Season, Gender, Temperature, Weight, Brightness, Motion
Anatomy and Physiology	Parts of the body Tissues and Organs Activity and Function
Pathology	Disorders, Pulses
Imbalances	Signs of Yang Repletion Signs of Yin Repletion

Yin-Yang Phenomena		
Phenomenon	**Yang**	**Yin**
Space	Heaven	Earth
Time	Day	Night
Season	Spring Summer	Autumn Winter
Gender	Male	Female
Temperature	Hot	Cold
Weight	Light	Heavy
Brightness	Radiant	Obscured
Motion	Upward and Outward Evident Motion	Downward and Inward Relative Stasis

Yin-Yang Anatomy and Physiology		
	Yang	**Yin**
Parts of the Body	Exterior, back, Upper body	Interior, abdomen, Lower body
Tissues and Organs	Surface skin Body hair Zang Organs	Bones Sinews Fu Organs
Activity, Function	Qi and Defense Agitation Strength	Blood and Construction Quietude Weakness

Yin-Yang Pathology	
Yin Disorders	**Yang Disorders**
Interior, Depletion, Cold	Exterior, Repletion, Heat
Yin Pulses	**Yang Pulses**
Slow, Deep, Rough, Deplete, Small, Fine	Rapid, Floating, Slippery, Replete, Large, Surging

1.2 Yin-Yang imbalances

Yin and yang are general categorizations underlying all other, more specific differentiations in Chinese medical diagnosis. In addition to general, overall signs of yin and yang patterns, there are patterns specific to body areas. It is essential, therefore, when first examining a patient, to note whether he or she presents a predominance of one or the other aspect.

Keep in mind that an excess, or repletion, of yang implies an insufficiency, or depletion, of yin, and vice versa, a phenomenon generally characteristic of acute conditions.

For example, an acute febrile disorder with fever, thirst, and perhaps constipation, represents a repletion of yang, which would be accompanied by a concurrent depletion of yin body fluids. However, in chronic conditions it is usual for a depletion of one aspect to cause an *apparent* repletion of its opposite aspect. The most common example is kidney yin depletion, a chronic condition often resulting in such apparent yang symptoms as ascendent hyperactivity of liver yang, heart and shen disturbances, etc. It is therefore essential to determine what is at cause (an initial repletion or an initial depletion), and to treat accordingly.

In extremely chronic conditions, many patients will present with a depletion of both yin and yang. In these cases, supporting either aspect will have a beneficial effect upon the other aspect. It is clinically impossible to have a mutual repletion of both yin and yang.

Signs of Yang Repletion	
Overall Yang Repletion	
Attitude	Self-confident attitude
Emotional	Aggressive, irascible
Muscle tone	Good muscle tone, firm tissues
Complexion	Ruddy complexion
Skin	Warm skin
Expression	Vivid expression
Eyes	Bright, lively eyes
Speech	Rapid speech, strong voice
Gestures	Rapid gestures
Stamina	Good physical and mental stamina
Circulation	Normal or exuberant circulation
Metabolism	Rapid metabolism
Sleep	Agitation, restlessness, insomnia
Illness Patterns	Acute conditions of sudden onset, high fever, spasms
Pulses	Right pulses generally stronger than left pulses Superficial pulses generally stronger than deep pulses Distal pulses generally stronger than proximal pulses
Upper Body Yang Repletion	
Primary Indicators	Warmth or sensation of warmth in head or face associated with cold feet
Pulses	Three upper limb yang channel pulses (LI, TB, SI) stronger than three lower limb yang pulses (ST, GB, BL)
Lower Body Yang Repletion	
Primary Indicators	Warm feet associated with a cool face
Pulses	Three lower limb yang channel pulses (ST, GB, BL) stronger than three upper limb yang channel pulses (LI, TB, SI)

Signs of Yin Repletion	
Overall Yin Repletion	
Attitude	Passive, apathetic, listless attitude
Emotional	Sadness, discouragement
Muscle Tone	Poor muscle tone, flaccid tissues
Complexion	Pallid complexion
Skin	Cold skin
Expression	Expressionless face
Eyes	Lackluster eyes
Speech	Slow speech, weak voice
Gestures	Weak gestures
Stamina	Easily fatigued mentally and physically
Sleep	Somnolence
Circulation	Circulatory stasis
Metabolism	Sluggish metabolism
Illness Patterns	Chronic conditions of long duration
Pulses	Left pulses stronger than right pulses Deep pulses stronger than superficial pulses Proximal pulses stronger than distal pulses
Upper Body Yin Repletion	
Primary Indicators	Pallor, hands colder than feet
Pulses	Three upper limb yin channel pulses (LU, PC, HT) stronger than three lower limb yin channel pulses (SP, LV, KI)
Lower Body Yin Repletion	
Primary Indicators	Extremely cold feet associated with a warm head or face
Pulses	Three lower limb yin channel pulses (SP, LV, KI) stronger than three upper limb yin channel pulses (LU, PC, HT)

2 Qi, Blood, Body Fluids, Essence

Qi, Blood, Fluids, Essence		
Qi	*Five Functions of Qi*	Activation, Warming, Defense, Transformation, Containment
	Fifteen Types of Qi	Prenatal, Postnatal, Cosmic, Grain, True, Correct, Evil, Organ, Channel, Construction, Defense, Ancestral, Center, Clear, Turbid
	Four Disorders of Qi	Qi Depletion, Qi Stagnation, Qi Counterflow, Qi Fall
Blood	*Three Aspects of Blood*	Governed by the Heart Stored by the Liver Managed by the Spleen
	Three Disorders of Blood	Blood Depletion, Blood Stasis, Blood Heat
Fluid	*Two Types of Fluid*	Liquid, Humor
	Four Disorders of Fluid	Damage to Liquid, Humor Desertion, Water Swelling, Phlegm-Rhuem (*tan-yin*)
Essence	*Four Types of Essence*	Congenital, Acquired, Reproductive, Essential

2.1 Qi

In Chinese Medical theory, qi refers to a range of dynamic physiological processes. Qi has five major functions in the human system.

Five Functions of Qi	
Activation	Qi is responsible for human growth and development, as well as all physiologic activity and metabolism.
Warming	Qi controls body temperature, allowing organs and tissues to function normally despite external environmental conditions.
Defense	Qi prevents exogenous pathogenic influences from entering the body, and if they do enter, it counters them to restore the body to health.
Transformation	Qi is responsible for the transformation of nourishment into blood and all bodily fluids, and their circulation and distribution throughout the body.
Containment	Qi prevents extravasation of blood and excessive loss of other body fluids, such as by oversecretion of sweat or excessive urination.

Differentiated into specific physiologic processes, qi is given different names according to the process it describes:

Fifteen Types of Qi	
Xiantian zhi Qi	**Prenatal** or congenital qi, inherited from one's parents; one's "constitution." Also known as *yuan qi:* origin, or source qi.
Houtian zhi Qi	**Postnatal** or acquired qi. Qi obtained from food and air.
Da Qi	**Cosmic** qi. Air or oxygen, as it is utilized in the body.
Gu Qi	**Grain** qi, also known as *shui gu zhi qi:* water and grain qi. Together with *da qi* constitutes *houtian zhi qi.*
Zhen Qi	**True** qi. The qi that fills and nourishes the body.
Zheng Qi	**Correct** qi. The defensive aspect of *zhen qi,* which protects the body from evil qi.

(Continued)

9

Fifteen Types of Qi *(Continued)*		
Xie Qi	**Evil** qi. Pathogenic or heteropathic qi. Refers to any external illness-causing factor, but usually to the six climatic factors.
Zangfu zhi Qi	**Organ** qi, the qi present in the *zang* and *fu* organs, maintaining their healthy function.
Jingluo Qi	**Channel** qi. Qi that flows in the channels and vessels (including blood vessels).
Ying (Rong) Qi	**Construction** qi. The yin aspect of channel qi. Qi that nourishes the blood, organs, and tissues.
Wei Qi	**Defense** qi. The yang aspect of channel qi. Qi that protects the blood, organs, and tissues.
Zong Qi	**Ancestral** qi. Respiratory qi (not "ancestral" in the sense of "prenatal," but rather as the precursor of all the other qi activity in the body).
Zhong Qi	**Center** qi. Middle burner qi, the qi of the spleen and stomach, which transforms food and drink. May also refer just to splenic qi.
Qing Qi	**Clear** qi. The subtle essence of food and drink, transformed by the spleen to nourish the body.
Zhuo Qi	**Turbid** qi. The dregs left over after clear qi is transformed from food. It descends through the gastrointestinal tract to be expelled as waste.

Qi manifests four primary patterns of disorder based on its physiological functions:

Four Disorders of Qi		
Disorder	**Causes**	**Characteristics**
Qi Depletion	Chronic illness, old age, weak constitution, malnutrition, taxation fatigue	General physical weakness, symptoms specific to depletion of each organ, for example: *Lung qi depletion* - shortness of breath, faint voice *Spleen qi depletion* - poor appetite, indigestion *Kidney qi depletion* - enuresis, seminal emission; defense qi depletion: aversion to wind, tendency to catch colds. *See section* **11.2** for detailed discussion of Qi Depletion Patterns.
Qi Stagnation	Emotional constraint, dietary irregularities, contraction of exogenous pathogens, trauma	Local pain, distention, feelings of oppression, painful distention of fluctuating intensity and nonspecific location
Qi Counterflow	Usually disturbances of the lung and stomach	*Lung qi counterflow* - cough, distressed and rapid breathing *Gastric qi counterflow* - nausea, vomiting, hiccough
Qi Fall	Splenic qi depletion	Dizziness, upper abdominal distention or depletion fullness, prolonged diarrhea, rectal or uterine prolapse

2.2 Blood (*xue*)

Blood is formed when the clear qi derived from the digestate of the stomach and spleen is passed into the lung where it is transformed into blood. Blood's main function is to nourish the entire body, including the skin, body hair, sinews and bones, channels and vessels, and all the organs and tissues.

There are three important physiological principles associated with blood, explaining how and where it is *governed*, *stored* and *managed*:

Three Aspects of Blood

Governed *by the heart*	This refers to the heart's function of pumping the blood throughout the entire body.
Stored *by the liver*	This refers to the liver's function of storing blood and maintaining patency of blood flow (i.e., preventing stasis).
Managed *by the spleen*	In Chinese medical theory, the containing power of the spleen is responsible for preventing the blood from "spilling out of the vessels" (i.e., hemorrhage).

Three Disorders of Blood

Disorder	Causes	Characteristics
Blood Depletion	Diminished blood production, profuse hemorrhage	Dizziness, palpitations, lusterless or withered, yellow, drawn complexion, colorless lips and tongue, fine pulse, insomnia, flowery vision, hypertonicity, dry skin, dry, lifeless hair *See section* **11.2** for detailed information about Blood Depletion Patterns
Blood Stasis	Qi stagnation or depletion, blood cold, blood heat, impact trauma	Dark, dull complexion, cyan-purple lips and tongue, stasis macules on tongue margins, thin or rough pulse *Secondary symptoms*: recurrent bleeding of purple-black or clotted blood, local hematoma (impact trauma stasis macules), essence-spirit disturbances
Blood Heat	Heat toxin entering the blood	Frenetic blood movement, hemorrhage (with bright red blood), maculopapular eruptions *Secondary symptoms*: restlessness, crimson tongue, rapid pulse, delirium, coma

2.3 Fluids

The term "fluids" embraces all normal fluid substances of the human body other than blood. Fluids are differentiated into two component aspects, **liquid** (*jin*) and **humor** (*ye*, also pronounced *yi*):

Two Types of Fluid	
Liquid	Fluids that are relatively thin, mobile, and yang in quality. Mostly found in the surface of the flesh and the mucous membranes. Liquids moisturize the flesh, skin, hair, eyes, ears, mouth, nose, and other orifices. Sweat and urine are produced from liquid.
Humor	Fluids that are relatively thicker, less mobile, and yin in quality. Located primarily in the *zang* and *fu* organs, the brain, and bones. Humors lubricate the joints and are partially responsible for lubricating the skin (sebum would be considered humor, while sweat would be considered liquid). Cerebrospinal fluid is an example of yin humor.

Four Disorders of Fluids		
Disorder	**Causes**	**Characteristics**
Damage to Liquid	Minor or temporary depletion of fluids due to fever, profuse sweating, heavy urination, vomiting, diarrhea	Thirst, dry, rough tongue fur, dry throat, lips, tongue, nose, and skin, dry, bound stool, short micturition with scant urine
Humor Desertion	As above, but far more pronounced. Usually a result of prolonged illness or later stages of exogenous heat illness	As above, but all more pronounced. Extremely poor general health, dry mouth, strong thirst, dry tongue, red or crimson in color, and peeled clean of fur
Water Swelling	Impairment of transformative action of lung, spleen, or kidney qi	Edemic swelling of the face, torso, or extremities
Phlegm-Rheum (Tan-Yin)	Usually impairment of pulmonary or splenic transformation; occasionally impairment of kidney qi transformation	Phlegm, cough, expectoration of white, foamy mucus (pulmonary or splenic transformation impairment); palpitation, rapid breathing, cough, copious expectoration of white, foamy phlegm, such as in cardiac failure or pulmonary edema (kidney qi transformation failure)

2.4 Essence *(jing)*

Essence is a primary element responsible for determining physical growth and development and maintaining life activity. It is the yin counterpart to yang "spirit" *(shen)*. The combination of essence and spirit, *jing-shen,* is used to denote vitality, both physical and mental. The careful reader will note the similarity, in definition at least, between certain types of essence and certain types of qi (for example between *Congenital Essence* and *Prenatal Qi*). It may be helpful to understand such parallels as reflecting different aspects of the same function, rather than as defining separate and distinct entities. Though somewhat oversimplified, essence may be understood as stored potential (Porkert calls it "unattached structive energy" in TFCM), while qi may be understood by its use and actualization ("configurational energy" according to Porkert).

Note that unlike qi, blood, and fluids, disorders of essence are not identified as separate clinical or theoretical entities. Disorders involving damage to essence are generally included in kidney pathology, or combined with other physiological constructs (such as "Essence-Spirit Disorders," which would be understood in relationship to the heart).

Essence may be differentiated into four types:

Four Types of Essence	
Congenital Essence	Prenatal essence, inherited from both parents, determining the individual's constitution, physical development, and, to some extent, lifespan.
Acquired Essence	Postnatal essence, acquired from food and air, and responsible for continued healthy function of the organism. It serves to supplement and reinforce the congenital essence.
Reproductive Essence	The reproductive ability in *both* men and women. Essence is stored in the kidney, and when the reproductive function becomes fully developed, this stored essence is transformed into reproductive essence, allowing the individual to produce offspring.
Essential (or essence) Qi	Essence that has been mobilized to maintain the functional activity of the organs.

3 Visceral Manifestation Theory: The Organs

Visceral manifestation theory encompasses not only the anatomy, physiology, and pathology of the major organ groups defined in Chinese medical theory, but also identification of specific illness patterns associated with each of those organs or organ groups.

The major internal organs in Chinese medicine are divided into *zang* and *fu*. Thus far, no suitable translation has been found to adequately represent these terms. *Zang* refers to the heart, lungs, liver, kidneys, and spleen — yin organs involved with the storage and transformation of vital substances in the body. *Fu* refers to the various bowels or bowel-like organs, the large and small intestine, the stomach, the gallbladder, and the urinary bladder. These are yang organs mainly involved in transporting nutrients into, or waste out of, the body. Various translations of these terms have included "solid and hollow organs," "organs and bowels," "viscera and bowels," "treasure and workshop organs" (Soulie de Morant), and even "depots and palaces" (Paul Unschuld, noting their historical reference). None of these translations really seem adequate; none really emphasizes the yin-yang, interior-exterior relationships of each of these organs in their paired groupings. Consequently, in the absence of a better translation, we have chosen to retain the terms *zang*-organs and *fu*-organs.

Organs will be studied in considerably greater detail in section **11.3**.

The Organs	
Zang Organs	Heart, Lung, Spleen, Liver, Kidney, Heart Governor ("Pericardium"- see note † on page 17, following.)
Fu Organs	Small Intestine, Large Intestine, Stomach, Gallbladder, Bladder, Triple Burner
Curious Organs	Brain, Marrow, Bone, Blood Vessels, Uterus, and Gallbladder (simultaneously considered a *fu* organ)
Zang-Fu Pairs	Heart - Small Intestine Lung - Large Intestine Spleen - Stomach Liver - Gallbladder Kidney - Bladder Heart Governor - Triple Burner

Zang Organs	
Zang Organ	**General Characteristics**
Heart	Governs the blood and blood vessels Regulates blood flow Stores the spirit Opens into the tongue Stands in interior-exterior relationship with the small intestine Expresses itself in the complexion The "Emperor" among the organs; the "supreme controller of the *zang-fu*"
Lung	Governs qi, controls respiration The "foundation of qi"; causes qi to descend Ensures regular flow through the water passages Governs surface skin and body hair Opens at the nose Expresses itself in the voice Controls *wei* qi and perspiration Aids the heart in blood circulation Stands in interior-exterior relationship to the Large Intestine The "High Minister" among the organs
Spleen	Governs movement and transformation of digestate Manages the blood (keeps it in the vessels) Controls fluid movement in stomach Sends clarified *qing* qi of digestate to the lungs Governs the muscles, flesh, and limbs Opens into the mouth, manifested in the lips Controls taste Controls the center: keeps the internal organs in their place Stands in internal-external relationship to the stomach The "Director of the Granary"
Liver	Stores blood Governs free-coursing of qi, bile secretion, and emotional activity Controls muscular, tendinous, and ligamentous activity Influences digestive function of the stomach and spleen Opens at the eyes Manifests in the fingernails and toenails Stands in internal-external relationship to the gallbladder The "general in charge of making plans"

(Continued)

Zang Organs *(Continued)*	
Zang Organ	**General Characteristics**
Kidney	Stores essence (*jing*) Controls birth, development, maturation Governs the bones and engenders marrow Reflected in the teeth Governs water metabolism Receives qi from the lungs; is the "root of qi" Maintains balance with the heart Opens into the ear and the "two yins" (anus and urethra) Reflected in the hair of the head Nourishes liver yin Stands in internal-external relationship with the bladder The root of the yin and yang of all the organs
Heart Governor ("Pericardium")	Protects the heart from exogenous pathogens Circulates yang qi of the kidney to the yin organs Activates, energizes, and controls the yin channels The "Minister of Leisure," as it creates feelings of joy or pleasure

In acupuncture theory, the so-called "pericardium" originally referred to in early acupuncture texts as the "heart-governor" or the "gate of life" *(ming-men)*, had nothing to do with the pericardial sac surrounding the heart. Pericardiac patterns, described below in section **11.9**, are in reality heart organ problems. This confusion has resulted from the attempts, since 1949, to reconcile acupuncture theory with traditional Chinese pharmaceutics, which did recognize the actual, anatomical pericardium as an organic entity. In classical acupuncture theory, however, the "heart-governor" is the yin aspect of the ministerial fire of the kidneys, the "mother of the yin channels," ultimately responsible for the production of construction (*ying*) and blood. To avoid confusion and maintain consistency with other texts, however, acupoints on the heart-governor channel will be identified throughout this text with the "PC" prefix.

Fu Organs	
Fu Organ	**General Characteristics**

Stomach	The "sea of nourishment," the "sea of water and grain"
	The "place of rotting and ripening of food"
	Separates the clear and turbid parts of ingested food;
	    sends the clear upward to the spleen, and the turbid
	    downward to the small intestine
	Normally sends qi downward
	Together with the spleen, is the root of post-natal qi

Small Intestine	"The official who receives abundance and transforms matter"
	Further separates the clear from the turbid in the digestate
	"Governs liquid": absorbs waste water, which is
	    transformed by kidneys into urine and conveyed to bladder
	Stands in external-internal relation with the heart (in
	    certain heart diseases one will urinate blood)

Large Intestine	"Controls transmission and drainage of dregs" Forms solid waste into stool before moving it out of the body Further absorbs fluid in waste, said to "govern humor" Large intestine channel controls the nose, throat, and teeth

Gallbladder	Stores and secretes bile
	The "Court of Justice," responsible for making decisions
	The "*fu* of internal purity": the only yang organ that
	    does not transmit an impure substance,
	    thus its simultaneous classification as a "curious organ"
	Gallbladder channel activates yang aspects of liver function

Bladder	Controls storing of fluid: receives, stores, and excretes urine Bladder channel activates yang aspects of kidney function The "Mandarin of a sub-prefecture," in the sense that it is responsible for storing and releasing at the proper time
Triple Burner	Refers to three specific body areas and their organs: *upper burner* (heart and lungs), *middle burner*, (spleen and stomach), *lower burner* (liver and kidneys). As such, it regulates the general ingestion, digestion, and egestion of food and fluids through the body Also refers to the water passages of the body; governs water metabolism by ensuring free flow of fluids through the water passages; has a general, overriding control on all the organs responsible for water metabolism Controls production of *wei* qi, transports essence or source qi from the kidneys to all the other organs via the source-*yuan* points (some sources say the well-jing points) of the channels

As with the heart governor ("pericardium"), the triple burner presents us with confusing, contradictory descriptions arising from the attempt to reconcile pharmaceutics with acupuncture. In pharmaceutics, the triple burner refers primarily to the "three burning spaces," and their associated organs, described above, and to food and fluid metabolism. In classical acupuncture theory, however, the triple burner is a *function*, the yang aspect of the ministerial fire, the "father of the yang channels," ultimately responsible for the production of *wei* and qi.

The Twelve Officials

Reflecting the social and political conditions of its time, the *Nei Jing* considered the twelve *zang-fu* organs to be in a hierarchical relationship with one another, and assigned them "ranks" that corresponded to various branches of the imperial government. These are often referred to as the "Twelve Officials." They are a convenient mnemonic device for remembering each organ's functional role in the body.

The Twelve Officials	
Lung	Controller of Receiving Pure Qi from the Heavens
Large Intestine	Controller of Drainage and Dregs
Stomach	Controller of Rotting and Ripening
Spleen	Controller of Transport and Transformation
Heart	Supreme Controller
Small Intestine	Official of Separating the Pure from the Impure
Bladder	Controller of the Storage of Water
Kidney	Controller of Water
Heart Governor	Official who Protects the Heart
Triple Burner	Official of Balance and Harmony
Gallbladder	Official of Wise Judgment and Decision Making
Liver	Controller of Planning

4 The Five Phases

Five Phase Theory extends the concept of the cyclic revolution of yin and yang through five distinct stages or movements, each qualitatively represented by the archtypical images of **wood, fire, earth, metal,** and **water**. These images represent the evolution of the seasons, the different stages of life, the different climates, etc. In Chinese medicine, each phase represents a paired *zang-fu* organ group, while the different five-phase cycles represent the different possible interactions between these organs and their related bodily functions, tissues, emotions, senses, etc.

Five-Phase Correspondences					
	Wood	**Fire**	**Earth**	**Metel**	**Water**
Yin Organ	Liver	Heart	Spleen	Lungs	Kidneys
Yang Organ	Gallbladder	Small Intestine	Stomach	Large Intestine	Urinary Bladder
Season	Spring	Summer	Late Summer	Autumn	Winter
Climate	Wind	Heat	Humidity	Dryness	Cold
Emotion	Discontent	Joy	Obsession	Worry	Fear
Sapor	Sour	Bitter	Sweet	Pungent	Salty
Cereal	Wheat	Millet	Rye	Rice	Beans
Meat	Chicken	Mutton	Beef	Horse	Pig (Sow)
Odor	Rancid	Scorched	Perfumed	Fleshy	Putrid
Color	Azure Blue	Red	Yellow	White	Black
Fluid	Tears	Sweat	Parotid Saliva	Sobs	Sublingual Saliva
Sense	Sight	Speech	Taste	Smell	Hearing
Number	Eight	Seven	Five	Nine	Six
Nourishes	Muscles	Vessels	Flesh	Skin	Bones
Flourishes in	Nails	Complexion	Lips	Body Hair	Hair
Direction	East	South	Center	West	North
Planet	Jupiter	Mars	Saturn	Venus	Mercury

The Four Cycles of the Five Phases	
Engendering	Each phase nurtures, produces, and benefits another specific phase, allowing its continued healthy function.
Restraining	Each phase restrains another specific phase, preventing it from becoming unduly powerful and causing harm.
Overwhelming	A pathologic condition wherein a particular phase is weakened to the point where the other phase that would normally restrain it "overwhelms" it instead, weakening it even further.
Rebellion	A pathologic condition wherein one phase becomes so disproportionately strong that it "rebels" against, and thus weakens, the phase that should normally restrain it.

Part II

Channels

The channels and connecting vessels are pathways that carry qi, blood, and fluids throughout the body. They are described in two main categories: **Major Channels** (primary channels), and **Connecting Vessels** (secondary or collateral channels).

In additional to the major channels and the connecting vessels, two categories of associated structures are also discussed: **Channel Sinews** (also known as "tendino-muscular meridians") and **Channel Divergences**.

Channels and Vessels	
The Major Channels	**12** Regular Channels **8** Irregular Vessels
The Connecting Vessels	**15** Major Connecting Vessels (*luo mai*) **Numerous** Reticular Connecting Vessels (*sun luo*)
Channel Sinews and Channel Divergences	**12** Channel Sinews (*Tendino-muscular meridians*) **12** Channel Divergences

5 The Major Channels

The major channels have clearly defined pathways that penetrate deep into the body. There are two types of major channels: the twelve regular channels and the eight irregular ("extraordinary") vessels.

The Major Channels	
The Twelve Regular Channels	Each has an organ to which it **homes** Each has an organ with which it **connects** Each is linked with another in an **interior-exterior pair** Each yin channel **communicates** with another yin channel, and each yang channel with another yang channel Each may be distinguished by its relative proportions of qi and blood
The Eight Irregular Vessels	They are employed in **coupled** pairs Each is accessed via a **master point**

5.1 The Twelve Regular Channels

The twelve regular channels are each related to a specific *zang* or *fu* organ, and are interconnected in a continuous flow of qi.

5.1.1 Distribution of the twelve regular channels

The twelve channels are bilaterally symmetrical. Each is identified in three ways:

— According to the limb along which it either originates or ends;

— According to one of the six divisions of yin and yang to which it corresponds; and

— According to its associated *zang* or *fu* organ.

Channel Distribution — Body	
Hand Channels	
Yin	**Yang**
Lung (*hand taiyin*)	Large Intestine (*hand yangming*)
Heart Governor (*hand jueyin*)	Triple Burner (*hand shaoyang*)
Heart (*hand shaoyin*)	Small Intestine (*hand taiyang*)
Foot Channels	
Yin	**Yang**
Spleen (*foot taiyin*)	Stomach (*foot yangming*)
Liver (*foot jueyin*)	Gallbladder (*foot shaoyang*)
Kidney (*foot shaoyin*)	Bladder (*foot taiyang*)

Note in the following table that the hand channels are yin-yang distributed anterior-posterior; foot channels are yin-yang distributed medial-lateral.

Channel Distribution — Limbs		
Hand Channels		
Position	**Yin** *(anterior)*	**Yang** *(posterior)*
Lateral	Lung (*hand taiyin*)	Large Intestine (*hand yangming*)
Midline	Heart Governor (*hand jueyin*)	Triple Burner (*hand shaoyang)*
Medial	Heart (*hand shaoyin*)	Small Intestine (*hand taiyang*)
Foot Channels		
Position	**Yin** *(medial)*	**Yang** *(lateral)*
Anterior	Spleen (*foot taiyin*)	Stomach (*foot yangming*)
Midline	Liver (*foot jueyin*)	Gallbladder (*foot shaoyang*)
Posterior	Kidney (*foot shaoyin*)	Bladder (*foot taiyang*)

The anatomical directions referred to here assume that the body is in standard anatomical position, with the arms at the sides, palm facing forward.

5.1.2 Interior-exterior relationships of the twelve regular channels

The yin and yang channels are paired in "interior-exterior" relationship. Interiorly, each channel "homes" to its associated organ and "connects" with its interior-exterior related organ. Exteriorly (on the body's surface), each yang channel has a corresponding yin channel, running more or less parallel to it on the opposite aspect of the limb or torso.

Channel Connections and Destinations		
Channel	**Homes To** **(Organ)**	**Connects To** **(Organ)**
Hand Taiyin	Lung	Large Intestine
Hand Yangming	Large Intestine	Lung
Hand Jueyin	Heart Governor	Triple Burner
Hand Shaoyang	Triple Burner	Heart Governor
Hand Shaoyin	Heart	Small Intestine
Hand Taiyang	Small Intestine	Heart
Foot Taiyin	Spleen	Stomach
Foot Yangming	Stomach	Spleen
Foot Jueyin	Liver	Gallbladder
Foot Shaoyang	Gallbladder	Liver
Foot Shaoyin	Kidney	Bladder
Foot Taiyang	Bladder	Kidney

Interior-Exterior Linkage of the Channels						
Interior	Lung	Heart Governor	Heart	Spleen	Liver	Kidney
	|	|	|	|	|	|
Exterior	Large Intestine	Triple Burner	Small Intestine	Stomach	Gallbladder	Bladder

5.1.3 Hand and foot channel communications

Hand and foot channels of the same name communicate with one another (*hand taiyin* with *foot taiyin*, etc.), the yang channels communicating uninterruptedly on the body's surface, and the yin channels internally via their related internal organs. These relationships can be extremely useful in treatment.

Channel Communications					
Hand Lung	Heart Governor	Heart	Large Intestine	Triple Burner	Small Intestine
|	|	|	|	|	|
Foot Spleen	Liver	Kidney	Stomach	Gallbladder	Bladder

5.1.4 Diurnal flow of qi through the channels: the "Chinese Clock"

Although qi and blood constantly flow through all the channels, each channel has a two-hour period when its qi and blood are at a maximum. This may be likened to a wave traveling through the regular channel system. It is said that it is easiest to drain (sedate) a particular channel when it is at its time of maximum qi, and easiest to supplement (tonify) it just after that time. Another theory states that it is best to supplement it during the period *opposite* it on the Chinese clock, i.e., twelve hours later, when its qi and blood would be theoretically at their lowest level.

GB
11PM-1AM

TB   LV
9PM-11PM   1AM-3AM

PC   LU
7PM-9PM   3AM-5AM

KI   **Diurnal Flow**   LI
5PM-7PM   **of Qi**   5AM-7AM

BL   ST
3PM-5PM   7AM-9AM

SI   SP
1PM-3PM   9AM-11AM

HT
11AM-1PM

5.1.5 Proportions of qi and blood in the regular channels

Classical theory from the *Nei Jing* (*Su Wen*, ch. 24) maintains that each of the channels has a particular proportion of qi and blood. This was considered of clinical significance when deciding whether to drain pathogenic repletion from a channel by needling to drain qi or bloodletting to drain blood.

Proportions of Qi and Blood in the Regular Channels		
Channel	**Proportions**	**Draining Method**
Taiyang (SI-BL)	More blood than qi	Bloodletting
Shaoyang (TB-GB)	More qi than blood	Needling
Yangming (LI-ST)	Replete with blood and qi	Needling or bloodletting
Taiyin (LU-SP)	More qi than blood	Needling
Shaoyin (HT-KI)	More qi than blood	Needling
Jueyin (PC-LV)	More blood than qi	Bloodletting

5.1.6 Pathologies of the major channels

There are two types of major channel pathologies: those associated with the external course of the channel, and those associated with its internal organ. Each major channel also has general signs of qi repletion or depletion. The fifteen major connecting vessels and the twelve channel sinews all have pathologies of their own.

5.2 The Eight Irregular Vessels

The eight irregular vessels are so named because they are not interconnected and do not have a continuous flow, serving rather as "reservoirs" that drain repletions or supply depletions in the regular channel system.

Each of the eight irregular vessels has a "master point," located on one of the twelve regular channels, which "opens," allowing qi and blood to enter or leave the channel. Two irregular vessels, the governing vessel (*du mai*) and the conception vessel (*ren mai*) have their own points, running up the posterior and anterior midlines of the torso respectively. The other six irregular vessels intersect with certain points on the twelve regular channels: these are known as "confluent points" and are essential in treatments utilizing the irregular vessels.

Irregular vessels are often used in pairs as "coupled" vessels, the function of one supplementing the function of the other.

Eight Irregular Vessels *(In Coupled Pairs)*	
Vessel	**Master Point**
Ren mai	LU-7
Yinqiao mai	KI-6
Du mai	SI-3
Yangqiao mai	BL-62
Chong mai	SP-4
Yinwei mai	PC-6
Dai mai	GB-41
Yangwei mai	TB-5

In the eight tables that follow, each irregular vessel is listed on the same page with the irregular vessel with which it is coupled.

Ren Mai *The Conception Vessel*	
Basic functions	"Sea of yin channels" (links bilateral yin channels, regulates their activity). Regulates menstruation, nurtures the fetus.
Main pathologic signs	*Repletion:* menstrual disorders and vaginal discharges, male urogenital disorders; head and neck pains; abdominal fullness, distention and pain; mouth and tongue abscesses. *Depletion:* Pruritis; heavy feeling in loins and lumbar area; *shan* (many kinds of abdominal pains, especially hernia - also called *shan qi*).
Connecting vessel	A connecting vessel separates from the primary channel at CV-15 and disperses downward over the abdomen. When this connecting vessel is replete, there will be abdominal stasis pain; when deplete, itching.
Important Points	Master Point: **LU-7** Master Point of Coupled Vessel: **KI-6** Points of Reunion with Coupled Vessel: **BL-1, CV-2**

Yinqiao Mai *The Yin Motility Vessel*	
Basic functions	Controls ascent of fluids and descent of qi, opening and closing of eyes, and regulates muscular activity in general.
Main pathologic signs	*Repletion:* General weakness of yang organs and functions with corresponding tension of yin organs and functions; aggravations that worsen at midday and improve by evening and at night (worst at sunrise); migraines, congestive headaches; contracture and spasm along yin channel-sinews of lower limbs (with corresponding flaccidity along lateral aspect); diurnal epileptic seizures; watery eyes, heavy sensation of eyelids or inability to open eyes, hypersomnia. *Depletion:* Aggravations during the night; nocturnal headaches, cramps, or convulsions; insomnia.
Important Points	Master Point: **KI-6** Master Point of Coupled Vessel: **LU-7** Xi-cleft Point: **KI-8** Points of Reunion with Coupled Vessel: **BL-1, CV-2** Confluent Points: **KI-6, KI-8, BL-1**

Du Mai
The Governing Vessel

Basic functions	"Sea of the yang channels" (links bilateral yang channels at GV-14, regulating their activity). Homes to the brain and connects to the kidney, affecting mental and reproductive functions. Traverses the spinal cord, affecting the spine, spinal nerves, and cerebrospinal fluid.
Main pathologic signs	*Repletion:* Opisthotonos, back pain and spinal stiffness, headaches; hallucinations, essence-spirit disorders; eye pains; hyperexcitability, seizures (e.g., epilepsy). *Depletion:* head slumps forward and feels heavy, walking with rounded shoulders; lack of physical and mental force, weakness of personality and character; hemorrhoids, sterility, impotence.
Connecting vessel	A connecting vessel leaves the primary channel at GV-1, forming two branches that ascend paravertebrally to the nape of the neck, where they then disperse over the head. When this connecting vessel is replete, there will be stiffness of the spine; when deplete, heavy-headedness.
Important Points	Master Point: **SI-3** Point of Reunion with Coupled Vessel: **BL-1** Master Point of Coupled Vessel: **BL-62**

Yangqiao Mai
The Yang Motility Vessel

Basic functions	This vessel is complementary in function to the yin motility vessel; thus its functions are complementary and opposite.
Main pathologic signs	*Repletion:* General depletion of yin organs and functions with corresponding tension of yang organs and functions; aggravations at the end of the day and at night; nocturnal crises, pains, and congestions; nocturnal epileptic seizures; dry and itching eyes; insomnia or restless sleep; contractions along yang channel-sinews of lower extremities (with corresponding flaccidity along medial side). *Depletion:* Fatigue, lassitude, weakness during the day; aggravations during the day that improve at night.
Important Points	Master Point: **BL-62** Master Point of Coupled Vessel: **SI-3** Xi-cleft Point: **BL-59** Confluent Points: **BL-62, BL-61, BL-59, GB-29, SI-10, LI-16, LI-15, ST-4, ST-3, ST-1, BL-1, GB-20.** Point of Reunion with Coupled Vessel: **BL-1**

Chong Mai
The Penetrating Vessel

Basic functions	"Sea of the twelve channels," "sea of blood" (regulates blood in the major channels). Particularly regulates menstruation and associated disorders.
Main pathologic signs	*Repletion:* Weakness of abdominal organs, menstrual block or irregularity, insufficient lactation, nervous or motor atony; impotence. *Depletion:* Lower abdominal spasms, contractures, and pain; prostatitis, urethritis, orchitis, seminal emission; metrorrhagia, menorrhagia, hematemesis (replete stomach and small intestine causes corresponding depletion in spleen and heart, which are unable to govern and contain blood).
Important Points	Master Point: **SP-4** Master Point of Coupled Vessel: **PC-6** Confluent points: **CV-1, ST-30†, KI-11, KI-12, KI-13, KI-14, KI-15, KI-16, KI-17, KI-18, KI-18, KI-20, KI-21.** †According to *Su Wen,* ch. 60. Point of Reunion with Coupled Vessel: **CV-23**

Yinwei Mai
The Yin Linking Vessel

Basic functions	Unites the yin major channels, reinforces and balances their respective flows, and generally regulates yin channel activity. Particularly affects construction (*ying*) and blood.
Main pathologic signs	*Repletion:* All deep pulses stronger than superficial ones; repletion of thoracic organs: heart pains, hypertension, delirium and nightmares, thoracic tightness and oppression, contracted feeling in lungs, dyspnea; with external depletion: weakness of homolateral shoulder, upper arm and hand, and weakness of contralateral lower extremity. *Depletion:* All deep pulses weaker than superficial ones; depletion of thoracic organs: timidity or fear, apprehension, nervous laughter, emotional depression; hypotension, weak respiration; with external repletion: pains in homolateral anterior shoulder, arm, and hand, pains in contralateral lower extremity.
Important Points	Master Point: **PC-6** Master Point of Coupled Vessel: **SP-4** Xi-cleft Point: **KI-9** Confluent Points: **KI-9, SP-12, SP-13, SP-15, SP-16, LV-14, CV-22, CV-23** Point of Reunion with Coupled Vessel: **CV-23**

Dai Mai
The Girdling Vessel

Basic functions	Binds up all channels running up and down the trunk, thus regulating upward and downward flow of qi in the body.
Main pathologic signs	*Repletion:* Superficial repletion of yang channels, lumbar and loin pain, pain in lower extremities; weakness of shoulders and upper extremities (opposite side); weakness of opposite eye, opposite breast, opposite ovary.
	Depletion: Cold or heavy sensation or weakness in loins and lumbar area; white vaginal discharge, uterine prolapse; inflammation and severe pains of opposite shoulder (impeding movement), upper extremity, eye, breast, or ovary; abdominal fullness and distention.
Important Points	Master point: **GB-41**
	Master Point of Coupled Vessel: **TB-5**
	Confluent points: **LV-13**†, **GB-26, GB-27, GB-28**
	†According to *Nan Jing*, ch. 3.
	Point of Reunion with Coupled Vessel: **GB-29**

Yangwei Mai
The Yang Linking Vessel

Basic functions	Unites the yang major channels, reinforces and balances their respective flows, and generally regulates yang channel activity. Particularly affects defense (*wei*) and qi.
Main pathologic signs	*Repletion:* General repletion of all yang channels: fever, headaches with heat symptoms, symptoms that worsen during violent weather (e.g., thunderstorms), pains or skin problems during weather changes; articular pains (especially in wrists and ankles); mumps; diarrhea.
	Depletion: Generalized coldness and lack of body heat; loss of energy and physical strength (especially during snowy or rainy weather).
Important Points	Master Point: **TB-5**
	Master Point of the Coupled Vessel: **GB-41**
	Xi-cleft Point: **GB-35**
	Confluent points (*Essentials*): **BL-63, GB-35, SI-10, TB-15, GB-21, ST-8, GB-13, GB-14, GB-15, GB-16, GB-17, GB-18, GB-19, GB-20, GV-16, GV15**
	(Porkert, citing the *Nan Jing* and the *Qi Jing Ba Mo Kao*): **BL-63, GB-35, TB-13, TB-15, LI-14, GB-21, SI-10, GB-20, GV-15, GV-16, GB-19, GB-18, GB-17, GB-16, GB-15, GB-14, GB-13, ST-8.**
	Point of Reunion with Coupled Vessel: **GB-29**

6 The Connecting Vessels *(luo mai)*

The connecting vessels serve to create secondary pathways of communication between the major channels, internal organs, and various tissues and areas of the body. As such, they complete the channel system, allowing it to penetrate every area of the body. There are two types of connecting vessels: the larger, major connecting vessels (*luo mai*), of which there are fifteen; and the smaller, reticular connecting vessels (*sun luo*) which are described in classical literature as "too numerous to count."

6.1. The Major Connecting Vessels *(luo mai)*

The fifteen larger, major connecting vessels (*luo mai*) consist of a vessel branching from each of the twelve regular channels, one each from the governing and conception vessel, and the so-called "great connecting vessel," which branches off the spleen channel at SP-21. The major connecting vessels are considered to follow a course superficial to the regular channels, and do not penetrate to the interior of the body. Although they have their own specific pathologies, they mainly serve to connect paired yin-yang channels, and are often used therapeutically when imbalance exists within paired yin-yang channels or their related organs.

The point where the major connecting vessels diverge from their associated channel is known as the *luo* point. It is often combined with the source (*yuan*) point of its paired yin-yang channel when treating yin-yang channel imbalances. This technique will be discussed further in section **8.4**.

6.2 The Reticular Connecting Vessels *(sun luo)*

The major connecting vessels themselves have hundreds of finer ramifications, known as reticular connecting vessels (*sun luo*), which serve to distribute qi and blood to literally every cell of the body. They are important theoretically, though they have no established clinical applications.

7 Channel Sinews and Channel Divergences

7.1 Channel Sinews *(the tendino-muscular meridians)*

Although often referred to as "Tendino-muscular meridians" (from the French *Traite de Medecine Chinoise,* by Dr. Andre Chamfrault), the term in Chinese is *jing jin,* literally translated as "channel sinews." Since, in literary Chinese, the modifier always comes before the word modified, this latter rendering is more accurate, and the *jing jin* must be thought of as "channel-like sinews," not as "sinew-like channels," as the former rendering would suggest.

Channel sinews, then, are groups of muscles, tendons, and ligaments that follow the paths of the twelve channels. They have no associated points, do not connect with internal organs, and all begin at the extremities of the four limbs. They do have their own pathologies, though mostly related to muscle and joint problems occurring along their course.

7.2 Channel Divergences

Channel divergences (also known as "distinct meridians," a term originating in the French works of Andre Chamfrault) are channels that branch off the major channels above the elbows and knees. They penetrate the interior of the body, linking up with their coupled interior organ. The yang divergences then reemerge to join their associated major channel, while the yin divergences link up with their coupled yang channels, flowing with them toward the head. This explains the effects of many yin channels on problems of the neck and head, although neither is traversed by yin channels. The symptomatology and treatment of channel divergence problems is ignored in modern texts; it belongs in the scope of the more classical, channel-oriented acupuncture techniques, and is thus outside the domain of this text. Non-Chinese readers are referred to *L'Energetique Humaine en Medecine Chinoise,* by Drs. Andre Chamfrault and Nguyen Van Nghi (Angouleme: Imprimerie de la Charente, 1969).

Part III

Points

An acupoint is essentially a weak spot along the course of a channel — a place where the activity of that channel may be more easily affected, whether by needles, moxa, or massage, than an adjacent area. The actual size of a point, judged by its effect on its associated channel and related organ and body areas, seems to differ according to location, but most points are considered to be only one to three millimeters in diameter. It would follow then, that the more accurately one can locate a point, the more effective one's treatment will be.

Different points have different characteristics, i.e., different effects on their associated channels and organs. Certain points are known to supplement or stimulate the channel, organ, or function; others seem to have a draining or calming effect. Still others seem to be homeostatic.

Although there is much disagreement about whether certain points supplement (tonify) or drain (sedate) certain channels, and even more disagreement on the techniques necessary to achieve these results, there is little disagreement on the relative importance of certain points on the body. Though there are other important categories of points outlined in the following pages, those considered most important are:

1) The **Five Transport-***shu* **Points** of the twelve major channels, all located between either the elbows and fingertips, or knees and toes;

2) The **Source-***yuan* and **Connecting-***luo* points, which act to reestablish harmony between paired yin-yang *zang-fu* organ groups;

3) The **Cleft-***xi* points, which have been found to be extremely effective in acute disorders; and

4) The **Back Transport-***shu* and (front) **Alarm-***mu* points, located on the posterior and anterior trunk, which seem to directly affect their associated organ.

Throughout the ages, specific therapeutic qualities have been ascribed to almost every point in the body. The best guide determining the use of these other, non-categorized points (mostly located on the trunk, upper arms and thighs, and head), is to palpate them for tenderness during the course of treatment. It is doubtful that a non-reactive point (with the exception of certain empirically determined points) will have much use therapeutically.

8 Point Types and Categories

17 Important Point Types and Categories	
Point Category	**Summary**
Transporting-*shu* **Points**	**5** points per per channel: also called "Antique;" important in five-phase applications.
Mother-Child Points	**1** Mother (supplementing) and **1** Child (draining) point for each channel.
Back Transporting-*shu* **Points**	**12** points, all on the back along the spine, each relating to a specific organ; also called "Associated" or "Assent" points.
Front Alarm-*mu* **Points**	**12** points, all on the torso, each relating to a specific organ; also called "Herald" points.
Source-*yuan* **Points**	**12** points, one per channel, each in direct communication with the channel's associated organ.
Connecting-*luo* **Points**	**15** points, one per each major channel (each the point of departure for the channel's connecting vessel) and one each for the Conception and Governing vessels, plus the "Great *luo* Point," SP-21.
Meeting-*hui* **Points**	**8** points, each with a therapeutic effect on a specific tissue group, region, or function.
Cleft-*xi* **Points**	**16** points, used in acute, painful or stubborn situations.
Master-*jiaohui* **Points**	**8** points, also called "confluent points," one for each of the eight irregular vessels; usually paired when used in clinical practice.
Lower Uniting-*he* **Points**	**6** points, each having a direct and powerful effect on an associated *fu* organ.

(Continued)

17 Important Point Types and Categories *(Continued)*	
Point Category	**Summary**
General Connecting-*luo* **Points**	**5** points (2 yang, 3 yin), affecting the Irregular Vessels, used to balance yin and yang; particularly effective before treatment.
Group Connecting-*luo* **Points**	**4** points, used to unite all the yin channels on the upper limbs, to unite all the yang channels on the upper limbs, and, similarly, to unite all the yin and yang channels on the lower limbs.
Command Points	**4** points, one each with a powerful effect on the abdomen, back, head, and face/mouth.
The Four Seas	**2** points each for the Seas of Nourishment and Marrow, **3** points each for the Seas of Qi and Blood.
Windows of the Sky Points	**5** points, each with a specific symptomatology relating to the inability of the yang qi to rise to the head.
Entry and Exit Points	**12** points, each connecting one channel to the next in the "Chinese clock" cycle (superficial circulation of qi) via a secondary vessel.
Intersection Points	Points where several channels cross. These are points where qi and blood easily become bound and congested; needling these points will have a beneficial effect on several channels at once (see table at section **8.15**).

8.1 The Five Transporting-*shu* Points

The five transporting-shu points are all found on the extremities, between the finger-tips and elbows or the toes and knees. They are some of the oldest points used in treatment, being mentioned in both the *Nei Jing* and *Nan Jing:* thus are they referred to as "Antique Points." Each of the five points has certain characteristics that make it useful in the treatment of specific disorders. In addition, each of the transporting points has a five-phase correspondence, which differs for the yin and yang channels. These correspondences are useful in determining supplementing and draining points according to the "mother-child" principle of five-phase theory.

Transporting-Shu Point Functions	
Classic of Difficult Issues	
Point	**Governs**
Well-Jing	Fullness below the heart
Spring-Ying	Body heat (fever)
Stream-Shu	Bodily heaviness and joint pain
River-Jing	Dyspnea, cough and alternations of cold and heat
Uniting-He	Counterflow qi and diarrhea

Seasonal Point Recommendations		
Inner Canon and the Classic of Difficult Issues		
Season	**Inner Canon**	**Classic of Difficult Issues**
Spring	Spring-ying	Well-jing
Summer	River-jing	Spring-ying
Fall	Uniting-he	River-jing
Winter	Well-jing	Uniting-he

Five Transporting-*shu* Points — Yin Channels					
	Points / Phase				
Channel	Well *jing* Wood	Spring *ying* Fire	Stream *shu* Earth	River *jing* Metal	Uniting *he* Water
Lung	LU-11	LU-10	LU-9	LU-8	LU-5
Pericardium	PC-9	PC-8	PC-7	PC-5	PC-3
Heart	HT-9	HT-8	HT-7	HT-4	HT-3
Spleen	SP-1	SP-2	SP-3	SP-5	SP-9
Liver	LV-1	LV-2	LV-3	LV-4	LV-8
Kidney	KI-1	KI-2	KI-3	KI-7	KI-10

Five Transporting-*shu* Points — Yang Channels					
	Points / Phase				
Channel	Well *jing* Metal	Spring *ying* Water	Stream *shu* Wood	River *jing* Fire	Uniting *he* Earth
Large Intestine	LI-1	LI-2	LI-3	LI-5	LI-11
Triple Burner	TB-1	TB-2	TB-3	TB-6	TB-10
Small Intestine	SI-1	SI-2	SI-3	SI-5	SI-8
Stomach	ST-45	ST-44	ST-43	ST-41	ST-36
Gallbladder	GB-44	GB-43	GB-41	GB-38	GB-34
Bladder	BL-67	BL-66	BL-65	BL-60	BL-40

8.2 Mother-Child Supplementation and Drainage Points

According to five-phase theory, "support the mother to nourish the child," i.e., if a certain phase is depleted, supplement the phase directly preceding it in the five-phase engendering cycle. Likewise, "drain the child to relieve the mother," i.e., if a certain phase is too replete, drain the phase directly succeeding it in the five-phase engendering cycle. Preceding-phase points are known as "mother points," and succeeding-phase points are known as "child points." Points on the affected channel may be chosen, and their effects may be additionally supplemented by adding the point of the same phase on the corresponding "mother" or "child" channel (see section **16.1**).

Mother-Child Points		
Channel	**Mother Point** *(Reinforcing)*	**Child Point** *(Draining)*
Lung	LU-9	LU-5
Large Intestine	LI-11	LI-2
Stomach	ST-41	ST-45
Spleen	SP-2	SP-5
Heart	HT-9	HT-7
Small Intestine	SI-3	SI-8
Bladder	BL-67	BL-65
Kidney	KI-7	KI-1
Heart Governor	PC-9	PC-7
Triple Burner	TB-3	TB-10
Gallbladder	GB-43	GB-38
Liver	LI-8	LI-2

8.3 The Back Transporting-*shu* Points and Alarm-*mu* Points

The back transport-*shu* and front alarm-*mu* points are points on the torso that directly affect a related *zang* or *fu* organ, despite the channel they are on. Traditionally, the back transport-*shu* points, being yang, were used for draining repletions, and the alarm-*mu* points, being yin, were used for supplementing depletions. Another theory holds that the yang back transport-*shu* points were best for treating the yin *zang* organs, while the yin alarm-*mu* points were best for treating the yang *fu* organs. Today, it is considered that back transport-*shu* points may be used for either supplementation or drainage of both *zang* and *fu* with good effect, although alarm-*mu* points are generally used for supplementation only. Moreover, corresponding back transport-*shu* and alarm-*mu* points are often combined with excellent effect.

Back Transporting-*shu* and Alarm-*mu* Points

Organ	Transport *shu*	Alarm *mu*	Scope of Treatment
LU	BL-13	LU-1	Respiratory system disorders such as cough, dyspnea, thoracic fullness and distention
PC	BL-14	CV-17	Heart illnesses such as cardiac pain and palpitations
HT	BL-15	CV-14	Heart and stomach disorders such as palpitations, stomach pain, and neurasthenia
LV	BL-18	LV-14	Liver and stomach disorders such as liver region pain, vomiting and regurgitation of acid fluid
GB	BL-19	GB-24	Liver and gallbladder disorders such as pain in the area of GB-24 and jaundice
SP	BL-20	LV-13	Liver and spleen disorders such as enlargement or pain in either organ, abdominal pain or distention, and poor digestion
ST	BL-21	CV-12*	Stomach region disorders such as stomach pain or distention and lack of appetite
TB	BL-22	CV-5	Water metabolism dysfunctions such as edema, ascites, and diarrhea
KI	BL-23	GB-25	Kidney and urogenital disorders, low back pain or soreness, seminal loss, and premature ejaculation
LI	BL-25	ST-25	Large intestine disorders such as constipation, diarrhea, and abdominal pain
SI	BL-27	CV-4	Small intestine, bladder and urogenital disorders such as gripping intestinal pain, *shan* qi, enuresis, urinary block, and seminal loss
BL	BL-28	CV-3	Bladder and urogenital disorders such as enuresis, urinary block, seminal loss, and menstrual disorders

* SI-7 is listed in some older texts as the alarm-*mu* point of the stomach.

8.4 Source-*yuan* and Connecting-*luo* Points

The source-*yuan* point of a channel is considered to be in direct communication with that channel's associated organ, and may be used for either supplementation or drainage. The connecting point of a channel is the point of departure for that channel's connecting vessel, and is used when there is an imbalance between paired yin-yang channels.

According to classical theory, when one paired channel is replete and the other is depleted, the connecting-*luo* point of the replete channel may be drained, or the connecting-*luo* point of the depleted channel may be supplemented. A later theory postulated that it was first necessary to determine which of the two channels was affected first (known as the "host" channel), and which one was subsequently affected (known as the "guest" channel). According to this "guest-host" rule, the source-*yuan* point of the "host" channel was combined with the connecting-*luo* point of the "guest" channel. If the "host" channel was depleted, causing repletion in the "guest" channel, the source-*yuan* point of the "host" channel would be supplemented, while the connecting-*luo* point of the "guest" channel would be drained. Conversely, if a repletion in the "host" channel caused a secondary depletion in a "guest" channel, the source-*yuan* point of the "host" channel would be drained, while the connecting-*luo* point of the "guest" channel would be supplemented.

Source-*yuan* — Connecting-*luo* Points			
Channel	**Points**		**Main Symptoms**
	Source *yuan*	Connecting *luo*	
Lung	LU-9	LI-6	Bronchitis, sore throat, shortness of breath, copious phlegm, perspiration, heat in the palms and soles, breast pain, shoulder pain that follows the lung channel.
Large Intestine	LI-4	LU-7	Throat and gum illnesses, lymph node inflammation in the neck, mumps, sore throat, dry mouth, yellow eyes, clear nasal discharge, nosebleed, and large intestine channel shoulder pain.

(Continued)

Source-*yuan* — Connecting-*luo* Points (Continued)			
Channel	**Points**		**Main Symptoms**
	Source *yuan*	Connecting *luo*	
Spleen	SP-3	ST-40	Stiff tongue, abdominal pain, bodily weakness and heaviness, constipation, jaundice, leg pain along the spleen channel, malarial illness.
Stomach	ST-42	SP-4	Nosebleed, facial numbness, stomach channel leg pain, malarial illness, abdominal distention, general weakness.
Heart	HT-7	SI-7	Heart pain, rapid heartbeat, dry mouth, yellow eyes, heart channel arm pain.
Small Intestine	SI-4	HT-5	Submandibular swelling and pain, shoulder pain, neck pain, deafness, arm pain along the small intestine channel.
Kidney	KI-3	BL-58	General weakness and lassitude, lack of appetite, decrease in visual acuity, lower back soreness, weakness in the lower extremities, grey facial color.
Bladder	BL-64	KI-4	Eye pain, neck pain, pain in the back, lower back or legs, epilepsy, psychiatric disorders, nosebleed, rectal prolapse, hemorrhoids, malarial illness.
Triple Burner	TB-4	PC-6	Deafness, sore throat, conjunctivitis, shoulder and back pain, intra-vertebral pain, constipation, urinary block, enuresis.
Heart Governor	PC-7	TB-5	Spasms or pain in the forearm or hand, chest pain, palpitations, nausea, restlessness, heat in the palms, incessant laughter.

(Continued)

Source-*yuan* — Connecting-*luo* Points (Continued)			
Channel	**Points**		**Main Symptoms**
	Source *yuan*	Connecting *luo*	
Liver	LV-3	GB-37	Testicular pain and swelling, *shan* qi pain, thoracic fullness, vomiting, abdominal pain, diarrhea, enuresis, urinary block.
Gallbladder	GB-40	LV-5	Pain in the chest and lateral costal region, headache, eye pain, malarial illness, enlarged thyroid, swollen lymph nodes in the neck.

8.5 The Eight Meeting-*hui* Points of the Eight Tissues

There are eight meeting-*hui* points, each of which has a therapeutic effect on a certain tissue, region or function. They may be added to any treatment dealing with problems associated with these particular functions or tissues.

The Eight Meeting-*hui* Points								
Point	LV-13	CV-12	CV-17	BL-17	GB-34	GB-39	BL-11	LU-9
Region of Effect	*Zang* Organs	*Fu* Organs	Qi	Blood	Sinews	Marrow	Bones	Vessels

8.6 Cleft-*xi* Points

Each of the twelve regular channels, plus the yinqiao, yangqiao, yinwei, and yangwei irregular channels, has a cleft-*xi* point, which is useful in treating acute, painful or particularly stubborn conditions. Cleft-*xi* points are often combined with the meeting-*hui* points, described above, to good effect.

The Cleft-*xi* Points							
Channel	LU	LI	ST	SP	HT	SI	BL	KI
	|	|	|	|	|	|	|	|
Point	LU-6	LI-7	ST-34	SP-8	HT-6	SI-6	BL-63	KI-5
Channel	PC	TB	GB	LV	Yangqiao	Yinqiao	Yangwei	Yinwei
	|	|	|	|	|	|	|	|
Points	PC-4	TB-7	GB-36	LV-6	BL-59	KI-8	GB-35	KI-9

8.7 Master-*jiaohui* Points of the Irregular Vessels

The master points of the irregular vessels have already been mentioned individually in section **5.2**. For convenience, they are presented here in table form, in their most frequently employed pairs.

Certain sources refer to these points as "confluent" points. A more precise translation of the Chinese *jiaohui xue* would probably be "points of intersection." However, this leads to confusion between these points, which do not actually intersect with the irregular vessels, and those points of the major channels that do. Thus, we have retained the older, more descriptive term "master points" for these points which, indeed, control their associated irregular vessel. We have reserved the term "confluent" for those channel points that actually intersect with the irregular channels.

The Master-*jiaohui* Points of the Eight Irregular Vessels		
Master Points	**Irregular Vessels**	**Regions of Effect** *(When Paired)*
PC-6 *SP-4*	Yinwei mai Chong mai	Heart, stomach, and chest
TB-5 *GB-41*	Yangwei mai Dai mai	Outer canthus, area behind the ear, shoulder, neck (front)
LU-7 *KI-6*	Ren mai Yinqiao mai	Diaphragm, throat, lung
SI-3 *BL-62*	Du mai Yangqiao mai	Inner canthus, neck (front and back), ear, shoulder, small intestine and bladder

8.8. The Six Lower Uniting-*he* Points of the Yang Channels

According to the classics, the uniting-*he* point of a yang channel has a direct, powerful effect on its associated *fu* organ. The three foot yang channels not only have their own uniting points, but they also have uniting points corresponding to the three hand yang channels, with which they are in direct communication. These six lower uniting-*he* points are used in treating illnesses of the six *fu* organs, and may be combined with the three upper uniting-*he* points of the three hand yang channels as well.

Because the yin channels begin at the feet, flow internally to connect with their associated and coupled yin organs, and then emerge externally to flow toward the fingertips, their "uniting points" are essentially internal. Thus, unlike the yang channels, which flow superficially from the fingertips to the toes, connecting with their associated internal organs via secondary vessels, the yin channels have no special pairs of uniting points.

The Lower Uniting-*he* Points					
Stomach	Large Intestine	Small Intestine	Gallbladder	Bladder	Triple Burner
ST-36	ST-37	ST-39	GB-34	BL-40	BL-39

8.9 The General *luo* Points

These are points affecting the irregular vessels that act on the general balance of yin and yang. They should be used at the beginning of a treatment session.

General *luo* Points	
Yang Points: TB-5, GV-1	*Yin Points:* PC-6, LU-7, CV-1

8.10 The Group *luo* Points

Each of these points unites the yin or yang channels of the upper or lower limb, governing the passage of qi and blood between these channels. They are used when all three channels are simultaneously disordered, and are particularly effective in correcting right-side / left-side or upper-body / lower-body yin-yang imbalances.

Group *luo* Points	
Three Arm Yang: TB-8	*Three Arm Yin:* PC-5
Three Leg Yang: GB-39	*Three Leg Yin:* SP-6

8.11 The Four Command Points

Each of the four command points has a powerful effect on a particular region of the body, and may be used as a principal point in the treatment of any disorder, internal or external, occurring there.

The Four Command Points			
Abdomen:	ST-36	*Back (upper and lower):*	BL-40
Head and Back of Neck:	LU-7	*Face and Mouth:*	LI-4

8.12 The Four Seas

The "four seas" are mentioned in the *Nei Jing* (*Su Wen*, ch. 33). They are the Sea of Nourishment, the Sea of Blood, the Sea of Qi, and the Sea of Marrow. Each has particular symptoms of repletion or depletion, with corresponding points that are supplemented or drained accordingly.

The Four Seas			
Sea	**Points**	**Signs of Repletion**	**Signs of Depletion**
Sea of Nourishment	ST-30, ST-36	Abdominal distention	Inability to eat
Sea of Blood	BL-11 (upper body), ST-37, ST-39 (lower body)	Sensation that the body has increased in volume.	General malaise, with inability to ascribe any particular cause.
Sea of Qi	CV-17, BL-10, ST-9	Chest pains, flushed complexion, dyspnea	Inability to speak
Sea of Marrow	GV-20, GV-16	Sensation of excess energy	Fatigue and cramps in the lower extremities

8.13 Windows of the Sky

According to the *Nei Jing* (*Ling Shu,* ch. 21), certain points may be needled when particular symptoms indicate that yang qi is unable to ascend to the head.

Windows of the Sky Points	
Points	**Symptoms**
ST-9	Severe headache, fullness in the chest, dyspnea
LI-18	Inability to speak (also bleed *jinjin* and *yuye*, M-HN-20, under the tongue)
TB-16	Sudden deafness, diminished visual acuity
BL-10	Severe muscular contractions and spasms, vertigo, feet cannot support the weight of the body
LU-3	Extreme thirst, nosebleed, blood ejection

Chapter 2 of the *Nei Jing Ling Shu* also includes CV-22, SI-16, SI-17, GV-16, and PC-1, but without offering associated specific symptomatologies.

8.14 Exit and Entry Points

Points that connect one channel to the next via a secondary vessel in the superficial circulation of qi (i.e., according to the "Chinese clock"— see section **5.1.4**) are termed entry and exit points. They are used, for example, when a stagnation in one channel causes a depletion in the succeeding channel. Supplementing a point of entry will supplement its channel; draining it will drain its channel. Supplementing a point of exit, however, will *drain* its associated channel. Thus, *both* the point of exit of the replete channel and the point of entry of the following depleted channel may be supplemented to reestablish the normal flow of qi. Note that not all points of entry or exit are the normal first or last points of their respective channels.

Exit-Entry Points											
Exit	LU-7	LI-20	ST-42	SP-21	HT-9	SI-19	BL-67	KI-22	PC-8	TB-22	GB-41	LV-14
	|	|	|	|	|	|	|	|	|	|	|	|
Entry	LI-4	ST-1	SP-1	HT-1	SI-1	BL-1	KI-1	PC-1	TB-1	GB-1	LV-1	LU-1

8.15 Points of Intersection

Channels intersect at certain points, usually via small secondary vessels. A point where two or three channels meet will have a strong therapeutic effect on all these channels, eliminating the need for using multiple points.

Intersection Points			
Point	**Intersecting Channels**	**Point**	**Intersecting Channels**
Bladder Points			
BL-1:	BL, ST, SI, *yinqiao, yangqiao*	*BL-33:*	BL, GB, LV
BL-11:	BL, GB, SP, LU	*BL-41:*	BL, SI
Liver Points			
LV-13:	LV, GB	*LV-14:*	LV, SP, *yinwei*
Gallbladder Points			
GB-2:	GB, TB, ST, LI	*GB-9:*	GB, BL
GB-4:	GB, ST, TB, LI	*GB-10:*	GB, BL
GB-5:	GB, ST, TB, LI	*GB-11:*	GB, BL, TB
GB-6:	GB, ST, TB, LI	*GB-12:*	GB, BL
GB-7:	GB, BL	*GB-14:*	GB, ST, LI, TB, *yangwei*
GB-8:	GB, BL	*GB-20:*	GB, TB, *yangwei*
Spleen Points			
SP-6:	SP, LV, KI	*SP-13:*	SP, LV, KI
Stomach Points			
ST-1:	ST, CV, *yangqiao*	*ST-8:*	ST, GB
ST-3:	ST, LI, *yangqiao*	*ST-9:*	ST, GB
ST-4:	ST, LI, *yangqiao*		

(Continued)

Intersection Points *(Continued)*			
Point	**Intersecting Channels**	**Point**	**Intersecting Channels**
Governing Vessel Points			
GV-1:	GV, LV, GB	*GV-20:*	GV, CV, SI, TB, LI, BL, GB, ST
GV-13:	GV, BL	*GV-24:*	GV, BL
GV-14:	GV, SI, TB, LI, BL, GB, ST	*GV-26:*	GV, ST, LI
GV-16:	GV, BL and *yangwei*	*GV-28:*	GV, CV, ST
GV-17:	GV, BL		
Conception Vessel Points			
CV-2:	CV, LV	*CV-12:*	CV, ST, TB, LU
CV-3:	CV, SP, LV, KI, ST, GB, BL, SI, TB, LI	*CV-13:*	CV, ST, SI
CV-4:	CV, SP, LV, KI	*CV-17:*	CV, SI, TB, SP, LV
CV-7:	CV, GB, HT, *chong*	*CV-24:*	CV, GV, ST, LI
Lung Points			
LU-1:	LU, SP	*LU-7:*	LU, CV
Large Intestine Points			
LI-20:	LI, ST		
Small Intestine Points			
SI-10:	SI, *yangwei*, *yangqiao*	*SI-18:*	SI, TB,
SI-12:	SI, TB, LI, GB	*SI-19:*	SI, TB, GB
Heart Governor Points			
PC-1:	PC, TB, LV, GB		
Triple Warmer Points			
TB-15:	TB, GB, *yangwei*	*TB-20:*	TB, SI, GB
TB-17:	TB, GB	*TB-21:*	TB, GB, SI

9 Points in Clinical Application

9.1 Point Formulae

Point Combinations for Systemic Applications	
To **strengthen the body's healing abilities** *during the course of any disease*	GV-4, GV-14, BL-18, BL-23, BL-43, CV-4, CV-6, ST-36, SP-6
To **stimulate gastrointestinal activity** *and improve absorption of nutrients*	BL-18, BL-20, BL-21, BL-25, ST-36, CV-12, ST-25
To **dissipate pulmonary congestion** *and generally supplement bodily function*	LI-11, LI-4, GV-14, BL-13, GV-12
For **colds, early stage febrile illness,** *and any other pattern that requires coursing or dissipating the exterior*	GB-20, GV-14, M-HN-9 (*taiyang*), LI-10, LI-11
To lower **blood pressure**	LI-14, LI-11, ST-36, PC-6
To **calm the spirit,** *clarify the mind, generally promote the flow of qi and blood, and to promote communication between yin and yang*	LI-4, LV-3 (*"Opening the Four Gates"*)
Any form of **insomnia**	HT-7, SP-6, LI-4, LI-11, ST-36, M-LE-5 GV-4, CV-6
Nausea *and vomiting*	LI-4, ST-36
All forms of **diarrhea** *and dysentery*	ST-36, SP-6, ST-25, BL-25, CV-8 (salt moxa), CV-4
General points for **wind** *pain*	CV-4, SP-6, ST-36
General wind-damp (rheumatic) **joint pain**	LI-11, ST-36
General preventive points to **strengthen resistance** *and to supplement bodily function*	CV-4, GV-12, BL-23, LI-11, TB-24 (*left*), ST-36, KI-3. Choose 3-6 points as appropriate.
Anemia, general blood supplementation	ST-36, SP-6, GV-14, BL-17, SP-10, GV-4, CV-6
External inflammation, sores, and swellings	LI-10, LI-11, SP-6

(From *Zhenjiu Linchuang Shouci*, pp. 105-106)

9.2 Points to Correct Improper Needling

Points to Correct Improper Needling		
Point	**Result When Improperly Needled**	**Correct With**
SP-6	Needled too deeply may cause emotional depression or faintness	ST-36
GV-11	Incorrect needling may cause sudden collapse	GV-1
GB-18	Incorrect needling may cause disorientation	BL-23
GV-22	Incorrect needling may cause sudden fainting when the patient stands up	BL-12
HT-7	Incorrect needling may cause mania	GV-6
CV-15	Needled too deeply may cause hiccough or shortness of breath	CV-12
CV-17	Incorrect needling may diminish the intellect	CV-22 (insert rapidly and do not retain)
LI-10	Incorrect needling may cause profuse bleeding	LI-5 (while applying finger pressure at LI-10)
GV-15	Incorrect needling may cause muteness	GV-26 (with vigorous stimulation)
GV-16	Incorrect needling may cause aphonia or shock	GV-26, CV-22
CV-8	This point should never be needled: doing so may result in testicular swelling	GV-4
CV-9	Incorrect needling may cause abdominal swelling	ST-25, KI-16
GB-21	Needling too deeply may cause thoracic oppression	ST-36

(From *Zhenjiu Linchuang Shouci*, p. 108)

9.3 Contraindicated Points

Contraindicated Points	
Point	**Comment**
GV-24	This point is now commonly needled .2-.3″
GV-17	Modern sources needle to .3″
BL-9	Currently needled .3″
BL-8	Currently needled .3-.5″
GB-18	Currently needled .3-.5″
TB-19	Currently needled .1″
TB-20	Currently needled .1″
ST-1	Currently needled .2-.3″; it can create a black eye - rarely used
GV-11	Some modern sources allow .5-1.0″ insertion here
GV-10	See GV-11
CV-17	Now needled to a depth of .3-.5″
LI-13	Sight of the radial collateral artery and vein
HT-2	Currently needled .3-.5″
CV-8	At the navel, forbidden to needle - salt moxa only
KI-11	Currently needled .5-.8″
ST-30	This is the site of a major artery; currently needled .3-.5″
SP-11	Currently needled .3-.5″; it is the site of a major vein and artery
BL-56	Some modern sources needle this point 1.0-1.5″
CV-9	Currently needled .5-1.0″. Should not be needled to treat water swelling (employ moxibustion)

(Continued)

<table>
<tr><td colspan="2" align="center">Contraindicated Points
(Continued)</td></tr>
</table>

Point	Comment
CV-1	Currently needled .5-.8 ″
ST-17	The nipple, forbidden to needle or apply direct moxa: use indirect moxa only
TB-8	Some modern sources needle this point .5-1.0 ″
LV-12	Site of femoral artery

<table>
<tr><td colspan="2" align="center">Contraindications in Pregnancy</td></tr>
<tr><td colspan="2" align="center">LI-4, SP-6, GB-21 and any abdominal points at any time during pregnancy;
8 liao (BL-31 through BL-34) during the first and second trimesters</td></tr>
</table>

9.4 Points with Opposite Effect Relationships

Points	Application	Point Effects
GB-34 / SP-10	Uterine bleeding	**GB-34** to stop bleeding **SP-10** to drain stagnant blood
GB-34 / SP-6	Vaginal discharge	**GB-34** to stop discharge **SP-6** to promote stagnant discharge
ST-34 / HT-7	Defecation	**ST-34** for loose stools **HT-7** for constipation
GB-34 / SP-6	Menstruation	**GB-34** to stop flow **SP-6** to promote flow
LI-4 / KI-7	Perspiration	**LI-4** (drained) to promote flow **KI-7** (supplemented) to stop flow
LI-10 / ST-36	Stomach activity	**LI-10** to speed up **ST-36** to calm down

(From *Zhenjiu Linchuang Shouci*, p. 61)

9.5 Important Points on the Ear

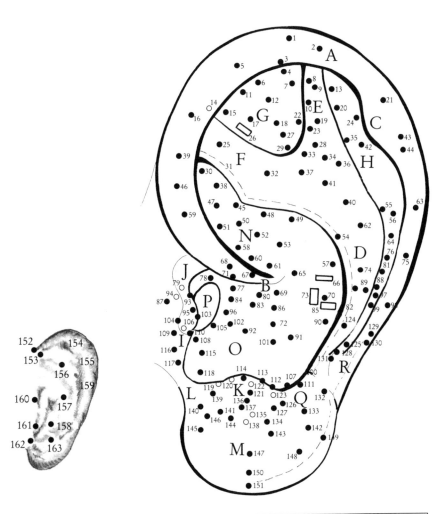

Key to Ear Geography			
A	Helix	**J**	Anterior Incisure
B	Crus of Helix	**K**	Antitragus
C	Auricular (Darwinian) Tubercle	**L**	Intertragic incisure
D	Antehelix	**M**	Lobule
E	Upper Crura of Antehelix	**N**	Cymba Concha
F	Lower Crura of Antehelix	**O**	Cavum Concha
G	Triangular Fossa	**P**	External Acoustic Meatus
H	Scaphoid Fossa	**Q**	Posterior Auricular Sulcus
I	Tragus	**R**	Tail of Helix

Note: These points indicate general locations only. Specific ear point locations should be confirmed by palpation or electronic detection.

Key to Ear Points

1 Ear Apex
2 Tonsil 1
3 Common Cold
4 Proximal Segment
5 Hemorrhoids
6 External Genitalia
7 Lower Blood Pressure
8 Heel
9 Toes
10 Ankle
11 Urethra
12 Uterus
13 Appendix 1
14 Sympathetic
15 Distal Segment Rectum
16 External Genitalia
17 Adnexa
18 Wheezing
19 Knee Joint
20 Fingers
21 Liver Yang 1
22 Neurogate
23 Gastrocnemius
24 Lesser Occipital Nerve
25 Sciatic Nerve
26 Constipation
27 Hepatitis
28 Hip Joint
29 Pelvic Cavity
30 Prostate
31 Sacrum
32 Buttocks
33 Popliteal Fossa
34 Knee
35 Allergy
36 Lower Abdomen
37 Heat Point
38 Bladder
39 Urethra (second one)
40 Lumbar Vertebrae
41 Abdomen
42 Wrist
43 Helix 1
44 Liver Yang 2
45 Ureter
46 Anus
47 Colon 1
48 Kidney
49 Pancreas/Gallbladder
50 Colon 2
51 Large Intestine
52 Ascites
53 Pancreas (second)
54 Lumbago

55 Abdominal wall
56 Elbow
57 Liver
58 Appendix
59 Distal Segment Rectum
60 Small Intestine
61 Duodenum
62 Abdomen
63 Helix 2
64 Appendix 2
65 Prolapse
66 Left Hepatomegaly Area
67 Nervous Dysfunction
68 Diaphragm
69 Stomach
70 Relax Muscles
71 Branch
72 Heart
73 Hepatitis Area
74 Thorax
75 Tonsil 2
76 Shoulder
77 Esophagus
78 Lower Abdomen
79 Thyroid 4
80 Pylorus
81 Axilla
82 Thoracic Vertebrae
83 New Eye
84 Mouth
85 Right Hepatomegaly Area
86 Upper Lung
87 Thirst
88 Shoulder Pain
89 Mammary Glands
90 Spleen
91 Lateral Lung
92 Bronchi
93 Tragus Apex
94 Throat
95 Clear Nose/Eyes
96 Trachea
97 Chest Wall
98 Helix 3
99 Shoulder Joint
100 Cervical Vertebrae
101 Lower Lung
102 Bronchi
103 Mid-Tragus
104 External Nose
105 Triple Burner
106 Inner Nose
107 Brain Stem
108 Upper Abdomen

109 Hunger Point
110 Adrenal
111 Thyroid 2
112 Vertigo
113 Brain
114 Parotid Gland
115 Bronchiectasis
116 Hypertension
117 Vision 1
118 Thyroid 3
119 Ovaries
120 Subcortex
121 Stop Wheezing
122 Testicles
123 Toothache
124 Neck
125 Clavicle
126 Throat & Teeth
127 Occiput
128 Thyroid 1
129 Tonsil 3
130 Helix 4
131 Appendix 3
132 Nephritis
133 Mandible
134 Vertex
135 Pituitary
136 Temple
137 Forehead
138 Emphysema
139 Vision 2
140 Raise Blood Pressure
141 Lower Palate
142 Maxilla
143 Upper Palate
144 Tongue
145 Neurasthenia
146 Tooth Extraction Anesthetic
147 Eye
148 Inner Ear
149 Helix 5
150 Tonsil 4
151 Helix 6
152 Superior Root of Ear
153 Spinal Chord 1
154 Lower Blood Pressure (Sup)
155 Lower Blood Pressure (Mid)
156 Lower Back
157 Middle Back
158 Upper Back
159 Lower Blood Pressure (Inf)
160 Vagus Root
161 Yang Linking
162 Inferior Root of Ear
163 Spinal Chord 2

Part IV

Pathology:
Causes and Patterns
of Illness

10 Causes of Illness

Illness may arise as a result of four general categories of causative factors: *exogenous* (environmental) causes, *endogenous* (emotional) causes, *independent* (lifestyle) causes, and what we have chosen to call the *additional* causes of *phlegm* and *static blood* (often classified separately).

Twenty Causes of Illness	
Six Exogenous Causes	Wind, Cold, Fire, Damp, Summerheat, Dryness
Seven Endogenous Causes	Joy, Anger, Anxiety, Preoccupation, Support, Fear, Fright
Five Independent Causes	Dietary Irregularity, Excessive Sexual Activity, Taxation Fatigue, Trauma, Parasites
Two Additional Causes	Phlegm, Static Blood

10.1 Exogenous Causes: The Six Environmental Excesses

The Six Environmental Excesses	
Wind	Rapid onset, swift changes in condition; convulsive spasm, tremor, shaking of head, dizziness, migratory pain, itching; invasion of upper body (esp. the head) and exterior (the lung, surface skin, and body hair).
Cold	Aversion to cold, desire for warmth, pronounced lack of warmth in extremities, cold and pain in lower abdomen; clear mucus, clear phlegm, watery vomitus, long micturition with clear urine, clear watery diarrhea; tendency to develop qi stagnation and blood stasis, severe pain; contracture and sinew-vascular hypertonicity or tautness; slow, tight pulse.
Fire	High fever, aversion to heat, desire for coolness, flushed complexion, reddening of the eyes, dark urine, red tongue with yellow fur, rapid pulse, pain, heat, swelling, red lesions; thick nasal mucus, thick yellow phlegm, sour watery vomitus, murky urine, blood and pus in the stool, acute abdominal diarrhea, foul-smelling stools, often with burning sensation on discharge. Damage to fluids: dry tongue, thirst with desire for cold fluids, dry hard stools. Hemorrhage, maculopapular eruptions, clouding of spirit-disposition, deranged vision, mania.
Damp	Physical fatigue, heavy cumbersome limbs, heavy head; aching joints, inhibited bending and stretching. Spleen symptoms such as: loss of appetite, indigestion, oppression in chest, heartburn, abdominal distention, thin stool, short micturition with scant urine, thick slimy tongue fur, soggy moderate pulse. Generalized, local stagnation of water-damp: water swelling, foot-qi illness (characterized by numbness of the legs, water swelling and heart disease, and corresponding to beri-beri), vaginal discharge, exudating lesions (e.g., eczema).
Summerheat	**Summerheat-heat:** high fever, thirst, restlessness, absence of sweating, surging pulse; weakness; short, distressed, rapid breathing; dry tongue fur. **Summerheat-damp:** remittent generalized fever, fatigued limbs, loss of appetite, oppression in chest, nausea and vomiting, abnormal stool, short micturition with dark urine, soggy pulse, thick slimy tongue fur.
Dryness	Dry nostrils, nosebleed, dry mouth, dry cracked lips, dry, tickly, or sore throat, dry cough with little or no phlegm, rough dry skin, dry tongue.

10.2 Endogenous Causes: The Seven Affects

The Seven Affects		
Affect	**Affected Organ**	**Symptoms**
Joy	Heart	Palpitations, racing of the heart, poor memory, insomnia, abstraction, sorrow, anxiety with tendency to weep, visceral agitation with frequent stretching and yawning. Manic agitation or essence-spirit derangement.
Anger	Liver	Essence-spirit depression, irascibility, pain in hypochondrium, eructation, globus hystericus. In women: breast lumps, painful distention of lower abdomen, menstrual irregularities.
Anxiety	Lung or Spleen	Melancholy, bitter depression of essence spirit, poor appetite.
Preoccupation	Spleen	Decreasing appetite, disturbed sleep, diminution of essence-spirit.
Support	Lung	Dejected, sorrowful countenance, pallor, lack of expression, easily saddened.
Fear	Kidney	Easily frightened, fearful of open places (prefers to stay indoors), overly cautious, easily disquieted.
Fright	Qi and Heart-Spirit	Emotional derangement, inappropriate speech and conduct.

10.3 Independent Causes of Illness

Five Independent Causes of Illness	
Cause and Examples	**Symptoms**
Dietary Irregularities: Ingestion of raw, cold, or unclean food. Voracious eating, overindulgence in fatty or sweet foods. Habitual consumption of alcohol or hot, spicy foods	Digestive disruptions, digestate accumulation, stomachache, diarrhea; may result in heat, phlegm, and damp.
Excessive Sexual Activity: Sexual overindulgence or giving birth to too many children	Wearing of kidney essence: lumbar pain, seminal emission, spiritual fatigue, general lack of strength, lassitude and dizziness. If from excessive childbirth: damage to penetrating and conception vessels, characterized by menstrual disruptions, menstrual block, vaginal discharge.
Taxation Fatigue: Refers to any harmful form of overexertion.	Frequently damages spleen, causing debilitation of original qi characterized by fatigue and weakness, lassitude of essence-spirit, yellow complexion, emaciation.
Trauma: Includes impact trauma, incised wounds, burns and scalds, snake bites.	————
Parasites: Includes blood flukes, roundworm, hookworm, pinworm, tapeworm	Similar to splenogastric damp-heat conditions

10.4 Additional Causes of Illnesses

Two Additional Causes of Illness		
Factor		**Symptoms**
Phlegm ...	*Congesting the lung*	Expectoration of large amounts of phlegm
	Lodging in the stomach	Nausea and vomiting
	Lodging in the channels	Subcutaneous phlegm nodules
	Confounding the cardiac portals	Spirit-disposition disturbances, coma
Static Blood		Localized pain, stasis macules, masses, hemorrhage, dull complexion, cyan-purple lips and tongue, stasis macules on edge of tongue, fine or rough pulse.

11 Patterns of Illness

Patterns of Illness	
Pattern Category	**Patterns**
Eight Parameter Patterns	Exterior and Interior Hot and Cold Repletion and Depletion Yang and Yin
Qi-Blood Patterns	Qi Depletion Patterns Qi Stagnation Patterns Qi Fall Patterns Qi Counterflow Patterns Blood Depletion Patterns Blood Stasis Patterns Blood Heat Patterns
Zang-fu Patterns	Heart (6), Lung (4), Spleen (3), Stomach/Spleen (4), Liver (10), Kidney (11) Stomach (3), Small Intestine (3), Large Intestine (2), Gallbladder (2), Bladder (2). *Numbers in parenthesis indicate number of patterns presented*
Pathogen Patterns	Wind, Cold, Heat and Fire, Summerheat, Damp, Dry, Digestate Accumulation, Phlegm.
Exogenous Heat Patterns	*Six-Channel Patterns:* Taiyang, Shaoyang, Yangming, Taiyin, Shaoyin, Jueyin
	Four-Aspect Patterns Defense (*wei*), Qi, Construction (*ying*), Blood
	Triple Burner Patterns Upper Burner (Lung and Pericardium) Middle Burner (Stomach and Spleen) Lower Burner (Liver and Kidney)
	Pericardiac Patterns Inward Fall of Pathogens to the Pericardium Clouding of the Pericardium by Phlegm Turbidity Stomach Heat Sweltering the Pericardium

11.1 The Eight Parameters

Eight-parameter pattern classification is the first and most important step in correctly determining the nature and location of an illness. The eight parameters are: **exterior and interior,** which determine the location of the disorder; **heat and cold,** which determine its thermic nature; **repletion and depletion,** which determine whether it is due to an exogenous pathogen or an internal weakness; and **yin and yang,** which generally classify the essential nature of the ailment itself. These factors provide the basic foundation upon which a more precise evaluation of the patient's condition can then be made. Eight-parameter patterns usually occur in combinations, outlined in the following tables.

Methods of Treatment have been included in the tables of Chapter 11 primarily as a study aid. These formally stated treatment methods, by concisely expressing the solution to a disease mechanism, often help define and clarify the nature of the mechanism itself. Noting, for example, that "cool, pungent exterior resolution" is employed in exterior heat patterns, while "diaphoretic exterior resolution" is employed in exterior cold patterns sheds additional light on the unique qualities of those two illness patterns, and brings their distinguishing signs and symptoms into sharper focus.

It is important to note, however, that many of these treatment methods are derived from herbal medicine applications. Although the history of acumoxa therapy in the west is often confused by the uneasy marriage between herbal medicine theories and acupuncture applications, the didactic advantages of their juxtaposition here, in our opinion, outweigh the disadvantages.

Exterior Patterns		
Pattern	**Principal Signs**	**Method of Treatment**
Exterior Heat	Mild aversion to cold; sore throat **Tongue:** Red body, thin, dry fur **Pulse:** Rapid, floating	Cool, pungent exterior resolution
Exterior Cold	Marked aversion to cold; headache; pronounced general pain **Tongue:** Thin, moist fur **Pulse:** Tight, floating	Diaphoretic exterior resolution
Exterior Repletion	No sweating **Pulse:** Tight, floating	Warm, pungent exterior resolution
Exterior Depletion	Sweating **Pulse:** Moderate, floating	Construction-defense harmonization

Interior Patterns		
Pattern	**Principal Signs**	**Method of Treatment**
Interior Heat	Red complexion or tidal flushing fever; aversion to heat; agitation; desire for warm beverages; short micturition with dark urine; hard, bound stool, or diarrhea with foul-smelling stool or blood in stool **Tongue:** Red or crimson with yellow fur **Pulse:** Rapid	Clearage
Interior Cold	Somber white complexion; aversion to cold and frigidity of the limbs; no thirst, or desire for warm beverages; abdominal pain relieved by warmth; long micturition with clear urine; thin or clear stool **Tongue:** Pale or white glossy **Pulse:** Deep, hidden or deep, slow	Warming
Interior Repletion	Abdominal fullness, distention with discomfort exacerbated by pressure; constipation; delirious mania **Tongue:** Thick, slimy, yellow fur **Pulse:** Deep, replete	Attack
Interior Depletion	Fatigue and lack of strength; shortness of breath; low voice; dizziness; flowery vision; palpitations; mental distraction; reduced appetite; thin stool **Pulse:** Fine, weak	Supplementation

Heat Patterns
(with Depletion and Repletion)

Pattern Type	Principal Signs	Method of Treatment
Repletion Heat (*Intense heat pathogen*)	Vigorous fever; restlessness and thirst; clouding of the spirit; delirious mania; abdominal fullness and distention with pain exacerbated by pressure. **Tongue:** Red with yellow fur **Pulse:** Fast, surging, slippery	Clear Heat and Drain Fire
Depletion Heat (*Yin humor depletion*)	Tidal fever; night sweating; emaciation; lack of strength; fever in the five hearts; dry throat and mouth. **Tongue:** Red tongue with little fur **Pulse:** Fine, rapid	Nourish Yin and Clear Heat

Cold Patterns
(with Depletion and Repletion)

Pattern Type	Principal Signs	Method of Treatment
Repletion Cold (*Cold pathogen congestion*)	Aversion to cold; cold limbs; cold and pain in the abdomen. **Tongue fur:** White, slimy **Pulse:** Deep, hidden, or tight, wiry	Warm and Free Repletion Cold
Depletion Cold (*Debilitation of Yang Qi*)	Aversion to cold; inversion frigidity of the limbs; drained white complexion; torpor of essence spirit; clear-food diarrhea; long micturition with clear urine. **Tongue:** Pale, enlarged, with thin, moist fur **Pulse:** Thin, slow, weak	Warm Yang and Restore the Correct

General Aspects of Depletion and Repletion Patterns		
Aspect	**Indicators**	
	Depletion	*Repletion*
Essence-spirit	Lethargy	Agitation
Bearing	Curled posture; desire for quiet	Flailing limbs
Complexion	Somber white, drained white, or withered yellow	Tidal flushing
Enunciation	Low	Strident
Speech	Little desire to speak or mussitation	Restlessness and talkativeness; delirious speech
Breathing	Shortness of breath	Rough
Chest and Abdomen	Depletion softness or pain and distention with intermittent relief	Hard, distended glomus with pain exacerbated by pressure
Pulse	Forceless	Forceful
Tongue Fur	Little or none	Thick and slimy

Repletion Patterns		
Qi Repletion Patterns		
Pattern	**Differentiation**	**Method of Treatment**
Lung Qi Repletion	Rapid dyspnea with copious phlegm, difficulty inhaling and exhaling (with sings of respiratory distress showing as straining of the mouth), inability to lie calmly	Drain lungs and transform phlegm
Stomach Qi Repletion	Abdominal distention, sour, fetid eructation, regurgitation of sour food, constipation or water diarrhea, bad breath	Adbuctive dispersal, harmonize the stomach
Blood Repletion Patterns		
Blood Repletion	Bumping and falling, abdominal distention and masses, menstrual block	Quicken the blood and disperse stasis; or disperse stasis and soften hardness
Internal Heat Repletion	Pulmonary swelling and purulence, fever with thirst, dyspnea, cough, and chest pains, purulent phlegm obstruction and effulgence **Tongue:** Red body, yellow, thick fur **Pulse:** Slippery, rapid, forceful	Clear heat and drain the lungs
Internal Cold Repletion	Intestinal spasms and contractions, and/or abdominal pain, patient tosses and turns, moans and groans, cyanotic complexion with frigid limbs **Tongue:** White, thick fur **Pulse:** Deep, tight, forceful	Warm the center and dissipate cold

Please note the format of the following table, a construction that will be used frequently throughout the book (particularly in section **11.3**). The signs and symptoms found directly beneath the title in these tables are those signs and symptoms *common* to all the patterns that follow them. The **Distinguishing Signs** that accompany each pattern in the body of the table should be used to differentiate those similar patterns.

Depletion Patterns		
Qi and Yang		
Drained white or somber white complexion; spiritual fatigue and lack of strength; spontaneous sweating; no energy to speak; low voice; non-transformation of ingested food; pale, enlarged tongue		
Pattern	**Distinguishing Signs**	**Method of Treatment**
Qi Depletion	Shortness of breath; lack of strength; rapid breathing at the slightest movement (all of these relatively pronounced); thin stool; dribbling incontinence **Pulse:** Soggy	Boost qi
Yang Depletion	Aversion to cold; inversion frigidity of the limbs; dark or cyan-purple complexion; long micturition with clear urine; clear food diarrhea **Tongue:** Cyan-purple **Pulse:** Slow	Warm yang
Blood and Yin		
Emaciation; dizziness; flowery vision; insomnia; palpitations; little tongue fur; fine pulse		
Blood Depletion	Pale white (or sallow) complexion; white nails; numbness of the limbs **Tongue:** Pale	Supplement the blood
Yin Depletion	Rising fire flush; fever in the five hearts; dry throat and pharynx; night sweating; seminal emission **Tongue:** Red or crimson, peeling or completely furless **Pulse:** Fine, rapid	Enrich yin

Yin and Yang Patterns		
	Indicators	
Aspect	*Yang Patterns, Repletion Heat*	*Yin Patterns, Depletion Cold*
Essence-Spirit	Manic agitation	Lethargy
Complexion	Tidal flushing	Drained white or somber white
Cold & Heat	Vigorous fever (or) no aversion to cold	No fever; frigidity of limbs; aversion to cold
Stool & Urine	Constipation and dark-colored urine	Clear urine and stool
Voice & Breathing	Rough breathing and strident voice	Shortness of breath; low voice.
Thirst & Drinking	Thirst; desire for cold beverages	No thirst; desire for warm beverages
Tongue	Red or crimson with yellow fur	Pale with white fur
Pulse	Rapid Slippery Replete Surging	Fine Soggy Faint Weak

Material for section **11.1** was translated from *Zhongyixue Gailun*, pp. 403-428

11.2. Qi-blood Patterns

Blood and qi are considered the fundamental constituents of the human body, and as such represent a more specific differentiation of the more general categories of yin and yang, described in section **11.1**. However, qi and blood themselves each differentiate into patterns of depletion and repletion, and certain organs may have specific qi or blood depletion or repletion patterns. Furthermore, the concepts of qi and blood as the two major aspects of physiologic function form the basis of the four-aspect pathogen penetration theory of the thermic illness school, described in section **11.6**. Following are the most usually encountered qi and blood patterns. Refer to sections **2.1** and **2.2** for summary information on additional illness patterns associated with blood and qi.

Common Qi Depletion Patterns	
Pattern	**Symptoms**
General Qi Depletion	*These symptoms accompany all manifestations of qi depletions:* General fatigue and lack of strength; devitalized essence-spirit; short, shallow breathing; no energy to speak; disinclination for physical movement; faint, low voice; spontaneous sweating; pale or enlarged tongue; soggy, forceless pulse.
Lung Qi Depletion	Cough and expectoration of phlegm in addition to relatively pronounced general symptoms such as: Short, rapid distressed breathing; no energy to speak; low voice.
Heart Qi Depletion	Slow, rapid or slow, irregularly interrupted pulse; palpitations or racing of the heart; disquieting of essence-spirit in addition to relatively pronounced shortness of breath; lethargy of essence-spirit.
Gastrosplenic Qi Depletion	Abdominal distention and oppression; indigestion; thin stool; center-qi fall; prolapse of the rectum and urinary frequency and urgency in addition to relatively pronounced withered yellow complexion, exhaustion of essence-spirit, and fatigued limbs.
Kidney Qi Depletion	Limp, aching knees and lumbar region; long micturition with clear urine; dribbling incontinence, enuresis, urinary block, and depletion of reproductive functions, together with a drained white or dull gray complexion, visual dizziness, mental clouding, tinnitus, deafness.

Common Blood Depletion Patterns	
Pattern	**Symptoms**
General Blood Depletion	*These symptoms accompany all specific blood depletions:* Lusterless or withered yellow complexion; mental dizziness; flowery vision; pale tongue; pale nails; fine pulse.
Heart Blood Depletion	Excessive dreaming and insomnia, in addition to the general blood depletion symptoms: palpitations or racing of the heart; poor memory.
Cardiosplenic Blood Depletion	*In addition to the general blood depletion symptoms and heart blood depletion symptoms:* loss of appetite; spiritual fatigue, menstrual irregularity, metrorrhagia, loss of blood.
Liver Blood Depletion	Dizziness; flowery or blurred vision; tingling in the limbs; hypertonicity of the limbs; dry nails; restless sleep; menstrual irregularity; amenorrhea or marked oligomenorrhea.

11.3. *Zang-Fu* **Patterns**

Each of the individual *zang* and *fu* organs may be affected, either by exogenous factors or endogenous damage. Each has its own characteristic pathologies of yin, yang, qi, or blood. Owing to their individual natures and functions, certain organs will tend more toward one type of disorder than another. For example, most liver disorders are characterized by either yang repletion, yin depletion, or a combination of both, but rarely is the opposite situation encountered (although an advanced cirrhotic state might be considered as such). Below are the major illness patterns of the *zang-fu* organs.

Zang-Fu Patterns	
Organ	**Potential Disorders**
Heart	Heart Qi Depletion Heart Yang Depletion Heart Blood Depletion Heart Yin Depletion Upflaming of Heart Fire Cardiac *Bi*
Lung	Non-Diffusion of Lung Qi Impaired Depurative Downbearing of Lung Qi Lung Qi Depletion Lung Yin Depletion
Spleen	Spleen Qi Depletion Devitalization of Splenic Yang Center Qi Fall
Stomach/Spleen	Blood Management Failure Gastric Qi Depletion Cold Insufficiency of Stomach Yin
Liver	General Binding Depression of Liver Qi Invasion of the Stomach by Liver Qi Hepatosplenic Disharmony Plumstone Globus Struma Disorders of the Governing and Penetrating Vessels Upflaming of Liver Fire Ascendant Hyperactivity of Liver Yang Liver Wind Liver Blood Depletion

(Continued)

Zang-Fu Patterns	
(Continued)	
Organ	**Potential Disorder**
Kidney	Kidney Yin Depletion Cardiorenal Yin Depletion Hepatorenal Yin Depletion Pulmorenal Yin Depletion Kidney Yang Depletion Splenorenal Yang Depletion Qi-Absorption Failure Cardiorenal Yang Debilitation Yang Depletion Water Flood Insufficiency of Kidney Essence Insecurity of Kidney Qi
Stomach	Stomach Heat Stomach Yin Insufficiency Stomach Cold Stomach Qi Depletion Epigastric Food Stagnation
Small Intestine	Depletion Cold of the Small Intestine Repletion Heat of the Small Intestine Small Intestine Qi Pain
Large Intestine	Large Intestine Repletion Heat Large Intestine Damp Heat Large Intestine Fluid Depletion Intestinal Depletion Efflux Desertion Large Intestine Depletion Cold
Gallbladder	Gallbladder Repletion Gallbladder Depletion
Bladder	Bladder Damp Heat Bladder Depletion Cold

Heart Illness Patterns *Depletion*		
Lusterless complexion; dizziness; palpitations; racing of the heart; shortness of breath; interrupted pulses		
Pattern Type	**Differentiation**	**Treatment Method**
Heart Qi Depletion	Shortness of breath; rapid breathing (from slight movement); essence-spirit fatigue; tendency to sweat. **Pulse:** Interrupted or slow, fine, weak **Tongue:** Pale, enlarged	Supplement heart qi; Nourish the heart and quiet the spirit.
Heart Yang Depletion	Dull grey or cyan-purple complexion; frigidity of limbs; yang depletion cold signs such as water swelling, cold sweating; heart qi depletion signs. **Tongue:** Dull, pale	Warm and free heart yang; Nourish the heart and quiet the spirit; In serious cases, salvage yang and secure against desertion.
Heart Blood Depletion	Dizziness; palpitations; racing of the heart; insomnia; poor memory. **Tongue:** Pale **Pulse:** Forceless, fine	Supplement the blood, boost qi; Nourish the heart and quiet the spirit.
Heart Yin Depletion	Dizziness; palpitations; racing of the heart; insomnia; upbearing fire-flush; restlessness; fever in the five hearts; night sweating. *Usually*: **Pulse:** Fine, rapid **Tongue:** Red	Enrich yin; Quiet the heart and spirit

Heart Illness Patterns
(Repletion)

Pattern Type	Differentiation	Treatment Method
Upflaming of Heart Fire	Cracked tongue; restlessness; red tongue tip In *breakdown of cardiorenal interaction* there may be insomnia, upbearing fire **Pulse:** Fast, fine pulse **Tongue:** Red, furless *Heart heat spreading to the small intestine* is characterized by painful strangury with dark-colored urine.	Drain heart fire Breakdown of cardiorenal interaction is treated by enriching yin and downbearing fire
Cardiac Bi	Stifling oppression and dull pain in the precordial region; paroxysms characterized by angina pectoris, cyan-purple complexion, cold sweat **Pulse:** Faint, fine, verging on expiry.	Perfuse heart yang Quicken the blood and transform stasis Transform turbidity

Lung Illness Patterns

Cough and rapid breathing

Pattern Type	Differentiation	Treatment Method
Non-Diffusion of Lung Qi	Usually occurs in acute paroxysms or is accompanied by exogenous contraction of exterior patterns. Dyspnea occurs when pathogenic heat or cold phlegm congests the lung.	Diffuse the lung
Impaired Depurative Downbearing of Lung Qi	Usually because of long-lingering pathogens. There is generally no exterior pattern.	Depurate and downbear lung qi
Lung Qi Depletion	Shortness of breath; thin, clear phlegm-drool; low voice and weak enunciation. **Tongue:** Pale **Pulse:** Deplete, weak	Supplement yang qi
Lung Yin Depletion	Dry cough; hoarse voice; dry mouth and pharynx; night sweating; emaciation; flushed cheeks; tidal fevers.	Enrich yin and moisten the lung

Splenic Illness Patterns
Splenic Transformation Failure

Fatigue; lack of strength; pale tongue

Pattern Type	Differentiation	Treatment Method
Spleen Qi Depletion	Lusterless complexion; diarrhea or thin stool; abdominal discomfort. **Pulse:** Soggy	Fortify the spleen and boost qi
Devitalization of Splenic Yang	Drained white complexion; abdominal pain relieved by warmth or pressure; clear-food diarrhea. **Pulse:** Deep	Warm yang and reinforce movement
Center Qi Fall	Emaciation; sagging and distention of the abdomen; bloating after eating. **Pulse:** Soggy	Fortify the spleen Upbear yang and boost qi

Spleen / Stomach Illness Patterns

Pattern Type	Differentiation	Treatment Method
Blood Management Failure	Hemorrhage (mainly hemafecia and metrorrhagia) occurring with: somber white or withered yellow complexion, lack of strength, shortness of breath. **Tongue:** Pale **Pulse:** Fine, soggy	Boost the qi and contain the blood Warm the spleen
Gastric Qi Depletion Cold	Epigastric pain relieved by pressure and eating	Fortify the center and warm the stomach
Insufficiency of Stomach Yin	Dry mouth; no thought of food or drink; depletion glomus of the epigastrium, retching. **Tongue:** Red mirror	Nourish stomach yin

Liver Illness Patterns
Binding Depression of Liver Qi

Pattern Type	Differentiation	Treatment Method
General Binding Depression of Liver Qi	Essence-spirit depression; painful distention of hypochondrium. **Pulse:** Wiry	Course the liver and rectify qi
Invasion of the Stomach by Liver Qi	Epigastric eructation; acid upflow; nausea; vomiting.	Course the liver and harmonizing the stomach
Hepatosplenic Disharmony	Abdominal pain; diarrhea, exacerbated by emotional factors.	Hepatosplenic harmonization
Plumstone Globus	Sensation of lump in the throat that can be neither swallowed nor brought up.	Downbear qi and transform phlegm.
Struma	Softer lumps either side of the throat that move up and down when swallowing.	Rectify qi and transform phlegm Disperse struma
Disorders of the Du mai and Yinwei mai	Irregular menses; painful distention of the breasts; breast lumps.	Regulate the governing and penetrating vessels

Liver Illness Patterns
Ascendant and Upflaming

Rashness; impatience; anger; headache; dizziness; red complexion; reddening of the eyes; dry mouth; wiry pulse; red tongue

Pattern Type	Differentiation	Treatment Method
Upflaming of Liver Fire	Sudden tinnitus or deafness; fecal block; rapid wiry pulse; rough yellow tongue fur.	Clear the liver and drain fire
Ascendant Hyperactivity of Liver Yang	Insomnia; palpitations; pain in the lumbar region; limp legs; rapid, fine pulse.	Enrich yin and calm the liver

Liver Illness Patterns *Wind Related*		
Pattern Type	Differentiation	Treatment Method
Liver Wind	Rigidity of the neck; tremor of the eyes, face, lips, and hands; inhibited speech; tingling numbness of the limbs; jerking sinews. *In serious cases:* convulsive spasms and tetanic inversion.	Calm the liver and extinguish wind Nurture yin and subdue yang
Liver Blood Depletion	Dizziness; flowery vision; scant menstrual flow; amenorrhea; insomnia; excessive dreaming; tingling numbness of the limbs; inhibited sinew-vascular movement	Nourish liver blood Enrich kidney yin

Kidney Illness Patterns *Yin Depletions*		
Dizziness; tinnitus; dry throat and lips; steady fever; pain in the lumbar region; seminal emission; fine, rapid pulse; red tongue		
Pattern Type	Differentiation	Treatment Method
Kidney Yin Depletion	(as above)	Enrich the kidney and nourish yin
Cardiorenal Yin Depletion	*All relatively pronounced:* Palpitations; insomnia; excessive dreaming; poor memory.	Enrich the kidney and nourish the heart
Hepatorenal Yin Depletion	Pronounced dizziness; headache; flowery vision; tinnitus.	Enrich the kidney and calm the liver
Pulmorenal Yin Depletion	*All relatively pronounced:* Dry cough; tidal fever; night sweating.	Enrich the kidney and nourish the lung

Kidney Illness Patterns
Yang Depletion

Dizziness; tinnitus; drained white complexion; spiritual fatigue; cold form; frigidity of the limbs; painful, limp knees and lumbar region; weak, soggy pulse; pale, fat tongue

Pattern Type	Differentiation	Treatment Method
Kidney Yang Depletion	Impotence; seminal efflux; sterility; polyuria and urinary frequency or nocturia.	Warm the kidney and restore yang
Splenorenal Yang Depletion	Persistent diarrhea or "fifth-watch" (5 A.M.) diarrhea.	Warm and supplement the spleen and kidney
Qi Absorption Failure	Dyspnea with distressed, rapid breathing; rapid breathing (at the slightest movement).	Warm the kidney and promote qi absorption
Cardiorenal Yang Debilitation	Water swelling; palpitations; dyspnea with rapid breathing; frigid limbs.	Salvage yang and secure against desertion
Yang Depletion Water Flood	Oliguria; water swelling; water-rheum intimidating the heart and shooting into the lung, characterized by palpitations and rapid breathing. **Tongue:** Pale, fat	Warm Yang and disinhibit water
Insufficiency of Kidney Essence	Diminished intellection; deficient reproductive function; hair loss; loosening of the teeth; poor development in children (soft bones, delayed closure of the fontanels).	Supplement the kidney and boost essence
Insecurity of Kidney Qi	Enuresis, polyuria; urinary frequency or incontinence; seminal emission or seminal efflux; low back pain; limp knees.	Secure the kidney and astringe essence

\multicolumn{3}{c}{**Stomach Illness Patterns**}
\multicolumn{3}{c}{*Counterflow Ascent of Stomach Qi*}
\multicolumn{3}{c}{Nausea, vomiting, eructation, or hiccups}
Pattern Type	Differentiation	Treatment Method
Stomach Cold	Exacerbated by cold, improved by heat, vomiting of clear fluids, desire for warm drinks, relief with pressure. **Tongue:** White, slippery or greasy fur	Warm the stomach and dissipate cold
Stomach Heat	Clamoring stomach, sour taste in the mouth, constipation; red urine; thirst with excessive consumption of fluids. **Tongue:** Red body with thick yellow fur **Pulse:** Rapid, slippery, forceful	Drain stomach fire
Stomach Yin Insufficiency	Dry mouth and lips; no appetite; hidden pain in the epigastrium, distention after eating; dry stool. **Tongue:** Red body with little fur **Pulse:** Fine and rapid	Enrich yin and nourish the stomach
Epigastric Food Stagnation	Epigastric and abdominal fullness with distention, resistant to pressure, regurgitation of putrid and foul smelling food or vomiting; distention relieved by vomiting, thin-stool diarrhea or bound stool. **Tongue:** Thick, greasy fur **Pulse:** Slippery	Disperse food and abduct stagnation; Disinhibit the *fu* organs and drain repletion
Stomach Qi Depletion	Epigastric fullness and oppression; no thought of food; frequent belching; clamoring stomach; bland taste in the mouth; loose stools; long micturition with clear urine. **Tongue:** Pale body with thin white fur **Pulse:** Depleted and weak	Reinforce qi and fortify the spleen

Large Intestine Illness Patterns		
Pattern Type	**Differentiation**	**Treatment Method**
Large Intestine Repletion Heat (Intestinal Heat Bind)	Dry mouth with parched lips, bound stool, distention and pain in the abdomen and umbilicus that is exacerbated by pressure; *or* watery, foul smelling stool; *or* pus and blood in the stool; feeling of urgency and heaviness in the rectum, or intestinal abscesses. **Tongue:** Dry, yellow fur **Pulse:** Rapid, replete	Clear heat and abduct stagnation
Large Intestine Damp Heat	Diarrhea with blood and pus in the stool; heavy sensation in the rectum; frequent but small bowel movements, nausea and vomiting, heavy sensation in the body with fatigued limbs, anorexic dyspepsia, burning sensation in the anus, short, red (dark) urination. **Tongue:** Red body with greasy fur **Pulse:** Wiry, slippery and rapid	Clear heat and transform damp to stop diarrhea
Large Intestine Fluid Depletion	Bound stool, only one movement every few days, vertigo, halitosis, dry mouth, parched throat. **Tongue:** Red body, dry coarse fur **Pulse:** Fine, rough	Enrich Yin and Nourish fluids; Moisten the intestines and disinhibit the stool
Intestinal Depletion Efflux Desertion	Chronic diarrhea, rectal prolapse; cold limbs; spiritual fatigue; diminished appetite; lusterless complexion. **Tongue:** Pale white **Pulse:** Depleted, fine	Strengthen the intestines to secure their containment ability
Large Intestine Depletion Cold	Thin stool or "duck-stool" diarrhea; abdominal pain and borborygmi; cold limbs and extremities; clear, extended urination. **Tongue:** Pale body with white, slippery fur **Pulse:** Deep and slow	Dissipate cold to check diarrhea

	Small Intestine Illness Patterns	
Pattern Type	**Differentiation**	**Treatment Method**
Depletion Cold of the Small Intestine	Hidden, intermittent pain in the lower abdomen relieved by warmth or pressure, abdominal distention, chronic diarrhea, thin stool diarrhea, borborygmi, frequent uncomfortable urination. **Tongue:** Thin, white fur **Pulse:** Slow or moderate	Warm and free the Small Intestine
Repletion Heat of the Small Intestine	Restlessness, agitation or heat in the cardiac region, thirst with desire for fluids; short, red, disfluent and painful urination. **Tongue:** Red body with yellow fur **Pulse:** Rapid and slippery	Clear and disinhibit repletion heat
Small Intestine Qi Pain (Repletion Cold)	Acute lower abdominal pain radiating to the lumbar and back; abdominal distention, borborygmi relieved by flatulence, *shan* pain in the scrotum. **Tongue:** White fur **Pulse:** Wiry	Move and dissipate binding

	Gallbladder Illness Patterns	
Pattern Type	**Differentiation**	**Treatment Method**
Gallbladder Repletion	Pain and fullness in the chest and hypochondrium; bitter taste in the mouth, sour retching, easily angered; little sleep but much dreaming; intermittent chills and fever; tinnitus; visual dizziness, vertigo. **Tongue:** Red, with yellow fur **Pulse:** Wiry, rapid, replete	Clear heat and disinhibit the gallbladder
Gallbladder Depletion	Bitter taste in the mouth, sour retching, fright, palpitations, anxiety; thoracic oppression; frequent sighing. **Tongue:** Thin, slippery fur **Pulse:** Wiry, fine and slow	Clear heat and transform phlegm; Downbear counterflow and harmonize the stomach

Bladder Illness Patterns		
Pattern Type	**Differentiation**	**Treatment Method**
Bladder Damp-Heat	Frequent, urgent, painful urination; urine may be turbid, bloody or calculous. **Tongue:** Yellow, greasy fur **Pulse:** Rapid	Clear heat, dissipate damp
Bladder Depletion Cold	Frequent urination which may be clear and extended, or urinary incontinence. **Tongue:** Pale with moist fur **Pulse:** Deep, fine	Secure containment of kidney qi

11.4 Pathogen Patterns

Illness patterns that result from the pathogens identified as the six climatic excesses, the dietary irregularities, phlegm, and blood stasis, are presented here as *Pathogen Patterns*. Distinguish these from the illness patterns caused by organ imbalance or dysfunction (called *Zang-fu Patterns*).

Pathogen Patterns	
Pathogen	**Potential Illness Pattern**
Wind	Contraction of Exogenous Wind Invasion of the Channels by the Wind Pathogen Wind Cold Damp *Bi*
Cold	Contraction of the Cold Pathogen Cold *Bi* Cold Pain Cold Diarrhea Cold *Shan*

(Continued)

87

Pathogen Patterns *(Continued)*	
Pathogen	**Potential Illness Pattern**
Heat and Fire	Repletion Heat Depletion Heat
Summerheat	Summerheat Heat Summerheat Damp
Damp	Damp Obstruction Damp-Heat Lodged in the Qi Aspect (in triple burner) Splenogastric Damp Obstruction Brewing Hepatocystic Damp-Heat Downpour of Damp-Heat into the Large Intestine Downpour of Damp-Heat into the Bladder
Dryness	Contraction of Exogenous Dryness Damage to Liquid Damage to Yin Blood Dryness
Phlegm	Damp Phlegm Cold Phlegm Heat Phlegm Wind-Phlegm Phlegm Confounding the Cardiac Portals Phlegm Lodging in the Channels or Limbs Phlegm Lodging in the Chest and Hypochondrium
Digestate Accumulation	Ingesta Damage Gastrointestinal Accumulation Splenic Depletion with Ingesta Damage Complication

Wind Illness Patterns		
Exogenous		
Headache; aversion to cold; fever; itchy throat; floating pulse		
Pattern Type	Differentiation	Treatment Method
Contraction of Exogenous Wind	**Wind Cold** — Pronounced aversion to cold with headache and aching bones or fever and thirst. **Tongue:** Moist, white fur	Warm, pungent exterior resolution
	Wind Heat — Unpronounced aversion to cold; sore pharynx; dry mouth. **Tongue:** Red	Cold, pungent exterior resolution
Channel Invasion		
Invasion of the Channels by the Wind Pathogen	**Local Sinews and Vessels** — Local palsy or paralysis	Dispelling wind and settling tetany
	General Sinews and Vessels — Rigidity of the neck; tetanus; convulsive spasm.	Dispelling wind and settling tetany
	Wind Cold Damp *Bi* — Muscular and articular pain	Dispel wind, transform damp, and dissipate cold

Cold Illness Patterns		
Pattern Type	Differentiation	Treatment Method
Contraction of the Cold Pathogen	Aversion to cold with: fever, headache, aching bones. **Pulse:** Floating, sometimes slightly tight. **Tongue fur:** Moist, white	Warm pungent exterior resolution
Cold Bi	Muscular or articular pain of relatively fixed location; Severe cases are characterized by hypertonicity.	Warm the channels and dissipate cold.
Cold Pain	Abdominal pain exacerbated by cold; history of cold contraction.	Dissipate cold and relieve pain
Cold Diarrhea	Abdominal pain and diarrhea relieved by warmth; lack of warmth in the extremities. **Tongue:** Pale with white fur	Warm the center and fortify the spleen
Cold Shan	Sagging testicles with pain reaching into the abdomen that is relieved by warmth. **Pulse:** Deep, wiry, tight **Tongue fur:** White, glossy	Warm the liver and dissipate cold Rectify qi and relieve pain

Heat and Fire Illness Patterns

Pattern Type	Differentiation	Treatment Method
Repletion Heat	Vigorous fever, restlessness, and thirst *In severe cases:* manic delirium; palpable heat and pain in the abdomen exacerbated by pressure; constipation or diarrhea with fetid stool, possibly containing pus or blood; maculopapular eruptions; hematemesis; epistaxis. **Pulse:** Slippery, rapid **Tongue fur:** Yellow	Clear heat and detoxify Drain fire
Depletion Heat	Tidal fever or inner-body fever; tidal flushing of the cheeks or upbearing fire, dry mouth and throat, steaming bone fever; night sweating. **Pulse:** Forceless, fine **Tongue:** Red with little fur or completely peeled fur	Enrich yin and clear heat

Summerheat Patterns

Pattern Type	Differentiation	Treatment Method
Summerheat Heat	Great heat; great thirst; profuse sweating or absence of sweating; agitation. **Pulse:** Large, surging	Clear summerheat
Summerheat Damp	Persistent low fever; lack of strength; thoracic oppression; nausea and retching; thin stool with feeling of discomfort after defecation; short micturition with dark-colored urine. **Tongue fur:** Thick, slimy	Clear summerheat and transform damp

Symptom Characteristics in Damp-Heat Patterns		
Symptom	Differentiation	
	When there is a prominence of damp	*When there is a prominence of heat*
Fever	Low, but generally persistent fever that is usually milder in the morning than in the evening	Higher fever
Chest and Abdomen	Discomfort, oppression	Pain, or painful and distention oppression
Thirst	No thirst, or thirst with no desire for fluid	Thirst and high fluid intake, or thirst with a desire for fluid and discomfort after drinking
Urine	Short micturition with scant, yellow urine	Short micturition with dark-colored urine
Pulse	Soggy, not too rapid	Slippery and rapid
Tongue	Slightly red tongue; slimy, white or dry, slightly yellow fur	Red tongue with thick, slimy, or rough, yellow fur
Treatment	Transforming damp, assisted by clearing-heat	Clearing heat, assisted by transforming damp

Damp Illness Patterns

Thoracic oppression; dyspeptic anorexia; upflow and nausea; sickly taste in mouth; abdominal distention; slimy tongue fur; general cumbersomeness and fatigue

Pattern Type	Differentiation	Treatment Method
Damp Obstruction	Low fever; repeated summer recurrence pattern.	Transform damp Dry damp Disinhibit damp
Damp-Heat Lodged in the Qi Aspect (in Triple Burner)	Fever; thirst with no desire to drink; short micturition with dark-colored urine. **Tongue fur:** Shiny yellow	Clear heat and transform damp
Splenogastric Damp Obstruction	Prominence of gastrosplenic signs; persistent fever is also possible. **Tongue:** Thick, slimy (possibly yellow)	(Pungent) opening and bitter discharge
Brewing Hepatocystic Damp-Heat	Jaundice; bitter taste in mouth; painful distention of chest and hypochondrium, possibly accompanied by abdominal pain; urinary frequency urgency, and turbidity **Pulse:** Rapid, wiry **Tongue fur:** Slimy (possibly yellow)	Course hepatocystic damp-heat
Downpour of Damp-Heat into the Large Intestine	Diarrhea with fetid stool (possibly with pus and blood); tenesmus, abdominal pain (possibly with fever); urinary frequency urgency, and turbidity	Clear heat and disinhibit damp Detoxify
Downpour of Damp-Heat into the Bladder	Urinary frequency urgency, and turbidity	Clear heat and disinhibit water Free strangury

Dryness Illness Patterns		
Dry mouth, dry lips, dry and bound stool		
Pattern Type	**Differentiation**	**Treatment Method**
Contraction of Exogenous Dryness	Dry cough; little phlegm; dry nose; epistaxis; blood in phlegm.	Clear the lung and moisten dryness
Damage to Liquid	Caused by high fever and excessive sweating. **Tongue:** Tends to be red with dry fur.	Engender liquid and clear heat
Damage to Yin	Usually occurs in latter stages of heat illnesses; generally poor physical state. **Tongue:** Clear with little fur **Pulse:** Fine, rapid	Enrich yin humor
Blood Dryness	Occurs in old age after prolonged nutritional disturbance or when static blood binds in the inner body. Signs include: general emaciation; rough, dry itching skin, thin, brittle nails, mirror tongue.	Nourish the blood and moisten dryness

Phlegm Illness Patterns

Cough; expectoration of phlegm; slippery pulse (possibly wiry)

Pattern Type	Differentiation	Treatment Method
Damp Phlegm	Copious, white, easily expectorated phlegm; thoracic oppression; fatigued, cumbersome limbs and other signs of spleen depletion damp encumbrance. **Tongue;** Thick, slimy fur	Dry damp and transform phlegm
Cold Phlegm	Thin, clear white phlegm; cold form; lack of warmth in the extremities. **Tongue:** Moist white fur	Warm and transform cold phlegm
Heat Phlegm	Thick, yellow phlegm possibly containing blood or pus; difficult expectoration; fever. **Tongue:** Red with yellow fur	Clear heat and transform phlegm

Slimy or unclean tongue fur, slippery pulse (possibly wiry)

Pattern Type	Differentiation	Treatment Method
Wind Phlegm	Sudden onset, foaming at the mouth, convulsive spasms.	Dispel wind phlegm
Upper-Body Harassment by Phlegm Turbidity	Dizziness (the major sign); thoracic oppression; nausea and slight vomiting, restlessness; bitter taste in the mouth	Transform phlegm and fortify the spleen Calm the liver and extinguish wind
Phlegm Confounding the Cardiac Portals	Sudden stupor of spirit-disposition, or essence-spirit derangement	Sweep phlegm and open the portals
Phlegm Lodging in the Channels or Limbs	Struma; phlegm nodules; scrofulous swellings or numbness of the limbs.	Disperse phlegm and soften hardness Free the connecting channels
Phlegm Lodging in the Chest and Hypochondrium	Distention and fullness in the chest and hypochondrium; pain caused by breathing or coughing; dyspnea with distressed rapid breathing; possibly facial edema.	Transform rheum and expel phlegm

Digestate Accumulation Patterns		
Thoracic oppression and bloating; little thought of food; slimy or unclean tongue fur		
Pattern Type	Differentiation	Treatment Method
Ingesta Damage	Nausea; vomiting; eructation of sour, putrid gas; painful abdominal distention; diarrhea or constipation; flatulence.	Abductive dispersion
Gastro-intestinal Accumulation	Hard abdominal glomus or abdominal pain exacerbated by pressure. **Tongue fur:** Old, yellow, or thick, slimy tongue fur.	Offensive precipitation
Splenic Depletion with Ingesta Damage Complication	Non-transformation of ingested food; thin stool or diarrhea with undigested food in stool; generally no abdominal pain. Tongue may be normal	Increase appetite and fortify the spleen Simultaneous dispersion and supplementation

11.5 Exogenous Heat Patterns

Exogenous heat illnesses are those characterized by fever in their early stages. They correspond to acute infectious illnesses in Western medicine, such as bacterial and viral infections, but also include forms of sunstroke.

There are two major systems, or schools of thought regarding exogenous heat illnesses: the "cold damage school," which maintains that both heat-induced and cold-induced exogenous illnesses penetrate via the six channels of the body, and the "thermic illness school," which maintains that heat-induced ("thermic") illnesses penetrate the body via the four aspects of wei, qi, ying, and blood. A third school of thought, developed in the Qing dynasty, maintains that certain illnesses, notably those of heat and dryness, penetrate the body via the "three burning spaces," i.e., the upper, middle, and lower burners.

Exogenous Heat Patterns	
Six-Channel Patterns	Taiyang, Shaoyang, Yangming, Taiyin, Shaoyin, Jueyin
Four-Aspect Patterns	Defense (*wei*), Qi, Construction (*ying*), Blood
Triple Burner Patterns	Upper Burner (Lung and Pericardium) Middle Burner (Stomach and Spleen) Lower Burner (Liver and Kidney)
Pericardiac Patterns	Inward Fall of Pathogens to the Pericardium Clouding of the Pericardium by Phlegm Turbidity Stomach Heat Sweltering the Pericardium

11.5.1 Six-Channel Patterns (The Cold Damage School)

Six Channel Patterns		
Pattern	Pathomechanism	Manifestations
Taiyang	Assailment of the exterior by wind cold	Exterior Repletion Exterior Depletion
Yangming	Gastrointestinal repletion heat	Channel Pattern Bowel Pattern
Shaoyang	Pathogen at midstage between exterior and interior	Exterior Pattern Interior Pattern
Taiyin	Gastrointestinal depletion cold	Like *yangming* bowel pattern but with signs of depletion
Shaoyin	Cardiorenal debilitation	Depletion Cold Depletion Heat
Jueyin	Interior depletion and cold/heat complex	Upper body heat with lower body cold

Taiyang Illness Patterns			
Aversion to cold or wind; general pain; fever; floating pulse			
Patho-mechanism	**Pattern Differentiation**		**Treatment Method**
Assailment of the exterior by wind-cold	**Exterior Repletion**	Absence of sweating; aversion to cold. **Pulse:** Tight	Warm, pungent exterior resolution
	Exterior Depletion	Sweating; aversion to wind. **Pulse:** Moderate	

Yangming Illness Patterns			
General fever; sweating; aversion to heat; restlessness; thirst			
Patho-mechanism	**Pattern Differentiation**		**Treatment Method**
Gastrointestinal repletion heat	**Channel Pattern**	Great fever; profuse sweating; great thirst. **Pulse:** Large, surging	Clear Heat
	Bowel Pattern	Tidal fever; delirious speech; abdominal fullness and distention with palpitation; tenderness; constipation. **Pulse:** Deep, replete, forceful	Offensive Precipitation

Shaoyang Illness Patterns

Alternating fever and chills, bitter fullness in chest and lateral costal region; vomiting; wiry pulse

Patho-mechanism	Differentiation		Treatment Method
Pathogen at midstage between exterior and interior	**Exterior Pattern**	Pain in the limb joints.	Harmonization
	Interior Pattern	Abdominal fullness and pain; constipation.	

Taiyin Illness Patterns

Abdominal fullness with intermittent pain; vomiting; diarrhea; no desire for food or drink; moderate, weak pulse

Patho-mechanism	Differentiation	Treatment Method
Gastrosplenic depletion cold	A digestive tract disorder like the *yangming* bowel pattern, but characterized by depletion rather than repletion.	Warm the center and fortify the spleen

Shaoyin Illness Patterns		
Patho-mechanism	Differentiation	Method
Cardiorenal Debilitation	**Depletion cold:** Aversion to cold; curled, recumbent posture; somnolence; inversion frigidity of the limbs; diarrhea. In serious cases: yang collapse depletion desertion. **Pulse:** Fine, faint	Salvage yang and check counterflow
	Depletion heat: Restlessness and insomnia; dry pharynx and mouth. **Pulse:** Fine, rapid	Enrich yin and clear heat

Note: Depletion cold is most common, though attention must be paid to the possibility of depletion heat.

Jueyin Illness Patterns		
Patho-mechanism	Differentiation	Treatment Method
Interior depletion and cold-heat complex	Upper-body heat and lower-body cold; diabetic illnesses; qi surging upward into the cardiac region; hunger with no desire for food; vomiting of roundworm; inversion frigidity of the limbs (occasionally).	Simultaneous warming and clearing

Note: It is important to determine the predominance of either cold or heat.

11.5.2 Four-Aspect Patterns (The Thermic School)

Four Aspect Patterns		
Pattern	**Pathomechanism**	**Differentiation**
Defense	Pathogen in the defensive exterior	Wind Thermia Damp Thermia
Qi	Exuberant heat in the qi aspect	First Stage Qi Aspect Heat Exuberant Pulmogastric Heat Great Heat in the Qi Aspect Gastrointestinal Heat Bind Heat Lodging in the Triple Burner Brewing Damp-Heat Steaming the Intestines and Stomach
Construction	Inward fall of pathogenic heat to the construction aspect	Inward Fall of Thermia Heat or Wind Thermia Inward Fall of Damp Thermia
Blood	Penetration of pathogenic heat to the blood aspect, causing depletion or frenetic blood movement	Repletion Heat at the Blood Aspect Depletion Heat at the Blood Aspect

Defense Aspect Illness Patterns			
Fever, slight aversion to cold or wind; headache; dry mouth, fast, floating pulse.			
Patho-mechanism	**Differentiation**		**Treatment Method**
Pathogen in the defensive exterior	**Wind Thermia**	Cough; sore, red pharynx. **Tongue:** Tends to be red	Cool, pungent exterior resolution
	Damp Thermia	General sensation of heaviness; thoracic oppression; upflow and nausea; dry mouth with no desire to drink. **Tongue fur:** Tends to be slimy.	Promote diffusion and transformation

Qi Aspect Illness Patterns		
Fever; aversion to heat rather than cold; thirst; bitter taste in the mouth; yellow or dark-colored urine; rapid pulse; yellow or mixed white/yellow tongue fur		
Patho-mechanism	**Differentiation**	**Treatment Method**
Exuberant heat in the qi aspect	**First Stage Qi Aspect Heat** — Thirst; restlessness. **Tongue fur:** Mixed yellow and white	Clear and outthrust pathogenic heat
	Exuberant Pulmogastric Heat — High fever, cough; rapid breathing; thirst. **Tongue fur:** Yellow	Clear heat and diffuse the lung
	Great Heat in the Qi Aspect — Great heat; great thirst; profuse sweating. **Pulse:** Large, surging	Clear qi with cold, pungent agents
	Gastro-Intestinal Heat Bind — Abdominal distention and oppression with pain exacerbated by pressure.	Flush accumulated heat
	Heat Lodging in the Triple Burner — Persistent, remittent general fever; thoracic oppression; upflow and nausea; thirst with no desire to drink; short micturition with scant urine. **Tongue fur:** Slimy, white or yellow **Pulse:** Soggy, rapid	Transform phlegm and clear heat
	Brewing Damp-Heat Steaming the Intestine and Stomach — Abdominal distention and oppression; hard, bound stool or diarrhea with fetid stool; **Tongue fur:** Slimy yellow **Pulse:** Deep, slippery, rapid	Dry damp and drain heat

Construction Aspect Illness Patterns

Red or crimson tongue, rapid pulse, general fever, restlessness, restless sleep. *In serious cases:* clouding of the spirit and tetanic inversion, or maculopapular eruptions

Patho-mechanism	Differentiation		Treatment Method
Inward fall of pathogenic heat to the construction aspect	**Inward Fall of Heat Thermia or Wind Thermia**	Red or crimson tongue with little or no fur	Clear construction
	Inward Fall of Damp Thermia	Crimson tongue with turbid or burnt black fur	

Blood Aspect Illness Patterns

Deep crimson tongue; maculopapular eruptions; hemorrhage; clouding of the spirit; convulsive spasm of the limbs; tetanic inversion

Patho-mechanism	Differentiation		Treatment Method
Penetration of pathogenic heat to blood aspect causing depletion or frenetic movement of the blood	**Repletion Heat at Blood Aspect**	Prominence of heat signs	Cool the blood and resolve toxin
	Depletion Heat at Blood Aspect	Pronounced signs of damage to yin	

11.5.3 Triple Burner Penetration

Triple Burner Pathogen Penetration	
Upper Burner	
Lung	Fever with either aversion to cold or sweating, headache, cough, thirst or lack of thirst, fever increases in afternoon. **Tongue:** Thin white fur **Pulse:** Floating, rapid
Pericardium	Spiritual stupor, delirious speech, agitation and thirst, disturbed sleep, limp tongue, inversion of limbs. **Tongue:** Red or crimson body **Pulse:** Fine, rapid
Middle Burner	
Stomach	Fever with no aversion to cold, sweating and thirst, constipation and difficult urination, other heat-dryness pattern signs. **Tongue:** Yellow, dry fur **Pulse:** Replete, large
Spleen	Generalized fever with inability to raise oneself, slightly worse in the afternoon, general feeling of heaviness, no thirst, oppression in chest, upflow and nausea, other damp-heat pattern signs **Tongue:** Thick, greasy fur **Pulse:** Soggy
Lower Burner	
Kidney	Generalized fever, flushed complexion, heat in palms and soles, restlessness and insomnia, cracked lips and dry tongue, scant, dark urine. **Tongue:** Red body with little liquid **Pulse:** Fine, rapid
Liver	Inversion in limbs (severe heat and severe inversion), vacant attitude but easily agitated, tremulous hands, in severe cases: chronic spasms. **Tongue:** Crimson body, little fur **Pulse:** Wiry, fine, rapid

11.5.4 Pericardiac Patterns

<table>
<tr><th colspan="3">Pericardiac Patterns</th></tr>
<tr><th>Patho-mechanism</th><th>Differentiation</th><th>Treatment Method</th></tr>
<tr>
<td>*Inward fall of thermic pathogens to the pericardium*</td>
<td>Coma or tetanic inversion; high fever; no pronounced changes in stool; no pronounced abdominal signs
Pulse: Rapid, and either fine or wiry
Tongue: Pure crimson with a fresh sheen; dry crimson with white fur or crimson with yellow-white fur</td>
<td>Portal opening (cool opening)</td>
</tr>
<tr>
<td>*Clouding of the pericardium by phlegm turbidity*</td>
<td>Coma or semiconsciousness; absence of high fever or non-vigorous surface fever; thin-stool diarrhea is sometimes observed; painful glomus and fullness; no pronounced abdominal signs.
Pulse: Rapid, and either soggy or slippery
Tongue: Slimy white fur covering the whole of the tongue or a turbid, slimy, yellow fur (tongue body is not necessarily crimson)</td>
<td>Portal opening (warm opening)</td>
</tr>
<tr>
<td>*Stomach heat sweltering the pericardium*</td>
<td>Delirious speech or manic agitation; late afternoon tidal fever or high fever; usually hard and bound, or diarrhea with fetid stool.
Pulse: Deep, slippery and forceful
Tongue: Thick, slimy, or yellow tongue fur</td>
<td>Precipitation (sometimes together with portal opening)</td>
</tr>
</table>

Part V

Diagnosis

Methods of Diagnosis	
Observation	Spirit Complexion Excretions Appearance Tongue
Audio-Olfaction	Listening Smelling
Enquiry	Chills and Fever Perspiration Thirst, Appetite, Taste Defecation and Urination Pain Hearing and Vision Sleep Menstruation and Childbirth History Emotions, Lifestyle, Home and Work Environment
Palpation	Pulse Examination Palpation of Channels and Points Abdominal Palpation

12 Observation

Method of Diagnosis	
Observation	Spirit Complexion Excretions Appearance Tongue

12.1 Observing the Spirit

Observation of the Spirit		
Characteristics	**Appearance**	**Indication**
Spirited	Bright eyes, normal behavior, keen responses, cooperative	Mild illness
Spiritless	Dull eyes, indifferent, sluggish responses, uncooperative	Serious illness

12.2 Observing the Complexion

Observation of the Complexion	
Appearance	**Indicates**
Lustrous, natural	Normal
Red	Heat
Pallor	Cold or blood depletion
Bright yellow	Yang jaundice
Cyan-purple	Blood stasis, severe pain

12.3 Observing the Excretions

Observation of Excretions	
Signs	**Indication**
Clear or white nasal discharge, sputum, urine, vaginal discharge	Cold or depletion
Turbid or yellow nasal discharge, sputum, urine, vaginal discharge	Heat or repletion

12.4 Observing the Appearance

Observation of the Appearance	
Physical Appearance	**Indications**
Obesity	Qi depletion, phlegm-damp
Emaciation	Depletion fire effulgence
Paralysis of limbs	Qi and blood depletion, channel obstruction
Convulsion, wry mouth and eyes, opisthotonos, twitching muscles	Yin and blood depletion causing malnutrition of tendons and vessels, or wind invasion of connecting vessels

12.5 Observing the Tongue

Observation of the Body of the Tongue	
Appearance	**Indications**
Pale	Depletion or cold patterns caused by weakness of yang qi, qi and blood insufficiency, or exogenous cold invasion
Red	Repletion or heat patterns due to exogenous heat invasion, or depletion patterns due to yin fluid depletion
Crimson	Severe stage of febrile illness: heat pathogen has passed into interior; or yin fluid exhaustion causing endogenous fire in prolonged illness
Purple (or purple spots)	Qi and blood stagnation; endogenous cold due to yang depletion
Large, flabby (pale, with teeth marks on border)	Qi and yang depletion, retention of phlegm-damp in interior
Red, flabby	Preponderance of heat pathogen in the interior, hyperactivity of heart fire
Cracked, fissured	Consumption of body fluid by repletion heat, kidney essence depletion, yin depletion fire effulgence
Thorny (red prickles)	Hyperactivity of heat pathogen
Rigid, tremulous	Exogenous heat invasion; phlegm confounding cardiac portals; liver yin depletion causing upstirring of liver yang; wind-phlegm obstructing the connecting vessels; in prolonged illness: qi and yin depletion
Deviated	Wind-phlegm obstructing the connecting vessels

Observation of the Fur of the Tongue	
Appearance	Indications
Thin white	Normal, or beginning invasion of exogenous wind-cold
Thick white	Food retention
Sticky white	Invasion of exogenous cold-damp; retention of phlegm-damp in interior
Dry white	Cold pathogen transforming into heat
Thin yellow	Wind-heat invading the lung
Thick yellow	Food accumulation in stomach and intestines
Sticky yellow	Accumulation of damp-heat in interior; phlegm-heat obstructing the lung
Dry yellow	Heat accumulating in stomach and intestines causing damage to yin
Moist grayish black	Retention of cold-damp in interior; endogenous cold due to yang depletion
Dry grayish black	Consumption of fluids by repletion heat; yin depletion fire effulgence
Peeled, glossy ("mirror tongue")	In a prolonged illness: major damage to correct qi, exhaustion of yin

13 Audio-Olfaction

Methods of Diagnosis	
Listening	Speech, Respiration, Cough
Smelling	Sputum, Urine, Breath

13.1 Listening

Diagnosis by Listening		
Object of Attention	**Characteristics**	**Indications**
Speech	Feeble, low tones	Depletion patterns
	Rapid, loud	Repletion patterns
	Delirious	Phlegm or heat confounding the heart
	Verbosity, mussitation	Mental derangement
	Stuttering	Wind-phlegm obstructing the connecting vessels
Respiration	Feeble breathing, shortness of breath, with sweating after slight exertion	Cardiopulmonary qi depletion
	Coarse breathing, asthma, frog-rattle	Phlegm-heat or phlegm-damp in the the lung
Cough	With course voice	Wind-cold invading lung; cold-phlegm accumulating in lung
	With clear voice	Wind-heat invading lung; phlegm-heat accumulating in lung
	Dry, little sputum	Dry pathogen injures lung; enduring lung yin depletion

13.2 Smelling

Diagnosis by Smelling		
Object of Attention	**Appearance**	**Indications**
Sputum	Thick, fetid	Phlegm-heat in the lung
	Dilute, clear, odorless	Cold-phlegm in the lung
Urine	Scant, dark, fetid	Damp-heat in the bladder
	Copious, clear, odorless	Depletion-cold in bladder
Breath	Malodorous	Stomach heat

14 Enquiry

Methods of Diagnosis	
Enquiry	Chills and Fever
	Perspiration
	Thirst, Appetite, Taste
	Defecation and Urination
	Pain
	Hearing and Vision
	Sleep
	Menstruation and Childbirth
	History
	Emotions, Lifestyle, Home and Work Environment

14.1 Enquire about Chills and Fever

Chills and Fever	
Symptoms	**Indications**
Simultaneous *when chills predominate* *when fever predominates*	Pathogenic invasion of exterior Wind-cold invasion Wind-heat invasion
Chills without fever	Endogenous cold from yang qi weakness, exogenous cold directly invades *zang* or *fu* organ
Sustained high fever	Exogenous heat pathogen replete in interior
Mild fever usually occurring in afternoon	Yin depletion
Periodic feverish sensation at body's surface conveyed from interior	"Steaming bone tidal fever"
Alternating chills and fever occurring at one, two, or three day intervals	Malarial illnesses

14.2 Enquire about Perspiration

Perspiration	
Symptoms	Indications
Sweating during exogenous pathogen invasion	Wind-heat invasion
Absence of sweating during exogenous pathogen invasion	Wind-cold invasion
Spontaneous sweating	Yang depletion
Night sweating	Yin depletion
Profuse cold sweating during severe illness	Yang qi desertion
Oily sweat	Breakdown of cardiorenal interaction

14.3 Enquire about Thirst, Appetite, Taste

Thirst	
Thirst Characteristics	Indications
Thirst with desire for cold fluids, high fluid intake	Interior heat patterns
Absence of thirst, or desire for warm fluids	Cold patterns
Thirst with little or no urge to drink; or immediate vomiting of fluids	Water-damp collecting in interior; impaired upbearing of fluids
Unallayed thirst with increase in urine volume	Diabetic illnesses

Appetite	
Food Preferences	**Indications**
Preference for cold food or beverages	Heat patterns
Preference for hot food or beverages	Cold patterns
Poor appetite, lack of taste in mouth, abdominal fullness	Splenogastric weakness
Disgust at sight or thought of food	Food retention

Taste in the Mouth	
Taste	**Indications**
Sticky, sweet taste	Damp obstruction; splenic depletion with damp
Bitter taste	Stomach heat; liver heat; hepatocystic damp-heat
Sour, putrid taste	Digestate stagnation
Intermittent acid upflow	Stomach heat; liver fire invading stomach

14.4 Enquire about Defecation and Urination

Patterns of Defecation		
Pattern	**Characteristics**	**Indications**
Constipation	Hard dry stool, fullness, pain, and distention in abdomen	Repletion and heat in the intestines (hot constipation)
	Hard stools with abdominal distention	Insufficiency of intestinal humor (cold constipation)
Diarrhea	Fulminant	Repletion
	Chronic	Depletion
	Shortly after eating	Gastrosplenic qi depletion
	Each day before dawn	Splenorenal yang depletion
	Frequent evacuation of small amounts of stool, with burning sensation	Damp-heat in large intestine
	Abdominal pain unrelieved by evacuation and brought on by emotional stimulae	Hepatosplenic disharmony

Patterns of Urination	
Characteristics	**Indications**
Deep yellow	Heat or repletion
Clear, profuse	Cold or depletion
Frequent, scant, deep yellow	Damp-heat accumulation in kidney and bladder
Frequent, clear	Depletion and cold in kidney and bladder
Urinary retention, difficult, dribbling urination	Damp-heat in bladder, kidney yang insufficiency, blood stasis, stones
Scant urination accompanied by water retention	Kidney and spleen depletion

14.5 Enquire about Pain

Pain: General Considerations	
Pain Characteristics	Pattern of Illness
Aggravated by pressure	Repletion
Alleviated by pressure	Depletion
Relieved by warmth	Cold
Relieved by cold	Heat
Migrating	Wind
Fixed	Cold-damp

Body Pains	
Symptoms	Indications
Pain over diaphragm	Heart and lung disorders
Pain in epigastric region	Spleen and stomach disorders
Pain in lumbar region or around umbilicus	Kidney and penetrating channel disorders
Pain below umbilicus and in lower abdomen	Kidney, bladder, intestinal disorders
Pain in costal and hypochondriac regions	Liver or gallbladder disorders

Headache Pain	
Characteristics	**Indications**
Occipital	Taiyang channels affected
Frontal	Yangming channels affected
Temporal	Shaoyang channels affected
Vertex	Jueyin channels affected
Recent onset	Exogenous illness
Prolonged	Endogenous illness
Severe	Repletion patterns
Dull	Depletion patterns
Exacerbated by exposure to wind and cold	Wind-cold disorders
Exacerbated by warmth	Ascendent hyperactivity of liver yang
Heavy-headedness, "bag-over-head" sensation	Phlegm-damp clouding upper body

14.6 Enquire about Hearing and Vision

Hearing	
Symptoms	**Indications**
Tinnitus, hearing loss	Depletion of kidney essence qi; shaoyang channel patterns; thermic illness repletion patterns
Gradual hearing loss in old age	Depletion

Vision	
Symptoms	Indications
Visual disturbance, flowery vision	Liver fire; ascendent hyperactivity of liver yang; hepatorenal essence-spirit depletion; blood depletion
Loss of visual acuity, dry eyes	Hepatorenal insufficiency

14.7 Enquire about Sleep

Insomnia	
Symptoms	Indications
Reduced, restless sleep, excessive dreaming, palpitations	Insufficiency of heart blood, disquieting of heart spirit, liver blood insufficiency
Restlessness, interior heat, inability to fall asleep, nightlong sleeplessness	Yin depletion fire effulgence
Persistent, severe, with both kidney and heart depletion signs	Breakdown of cardiorenal interaction
Gastric discomfort	Splenogastric depletion, phlegm-fire harassing upper body

Somnolence	
Symptoms	**Indications**
General lassitude	Depletion of heart and kidney yang
Lethargy with dizziness	Phlegm-damp accumulation in interior
Stupor with heat signs	Heat entering pericardium
Stupor without heat signs, but with sputum rattling; thick, sticky tongue	Phlegm confounding the cardiac portals

14.8 Enquire about Menstruation and Childbirth

Menstrual Patterns	
Indication	**Characteristics**
Blood Heat	Premature arrival, heavy flow, thick red discharge
Blood Depletion	Delayed arrival, reduced flow, light-colored discharge
Qi Depletion	Heavy flow, thin, light colored discharge
Blood Stasis	Purple, clotted discharge
Penetrating Vessel Disorder	Irregular periods and flow

Childbearing	
History	**Diagnostic Implications**
Excessive childbearing	Depletion of penetrating and conception vessels
History of miscarriage or difficult delivery	Insufficiency of qi and blood; hepatorenal depletion

Vaginal Discharges	
Symptoms	Indications
White, watery, little odor accompanied by backache	Spleen and kidney yang depletion; endogenous cold accumulation
Thick, yellow, fetid	Downward flowing of damp-heat
Irregular uterine bleeding after menopause; pus or blood mixed in discharge	Damp toxin in uterus

14.9 Enquire about the History of the Disorder

Presence of persistent, chronic ailments: An accident or past trauma may cause a predisposition to certain ailments. In addition, surgeries may cause blockage or stagnation in the acupuncture channels affected.

Previous treatments and medications: Efficacy or failure of previous treatments or medications used by the patient may give valuable information regarding the nature of the disease. Toxicity from allopathic medications should also be taken into consideration.

14.10 Enquire about Emotions, Lifestyle, Home and Work Environment

Emotional Attitude	
Characteristics	Indications
Taciturn and melancholy	Prone to binding depression of liver qi
Impulsive, rash, impatient	Upflaming of liver fire; upstirring of liver yang

Lifestyle: A prediliction for cold, raw, or fatty foods, or for smoking tobacco , indicates a tendency to phlegm-damp.

Home and work environment: Determine if stress level both at home and at work is mild, moderate, or heavy. In addition, attention should be paid to diseases commonly associated with certain occupations.

15 Palpation

Methods of Diagnosis	
Palpation	Pulse Examination Palpation of Channels and Points Abdominal Palpation

15.1 Radial Pulse Positions

Radial Pulse Positions and Correspondences			
Radial Position	**Depth**	**Left Side**	**Right Side**
After the Nei Jing (Su Wen, 17:7), circa 200-100 B.C.			
Inch (Distal)	*Superficial*	Left Thorax	Right Chest
	Deep	Heart	Lungs
Barrier (Middle)	*Superficial*	Diaphragm	Spleen
	Deep	Liver	Stomach
Foot (Proximal)	*Superficial*	Abdomen	Abdomen
	Deep	Kidney	Kidney
After the Nan Jing (ch. 18), circa 200 A.D.			
Inch (Distal)	*Superficial*	Hand taiyang	Hand yangming
	Deep	Hand shaoyin	Hand taiyin
Barrier (Middle)	*Superficial*	Leg shaoyang	Leg yangming
	Deep	Leg jueyin	Leg taiyin
Foot (Proximal)	*Superficial*	Leg taiyang	Hand shaoyang
	Deep	Leg shaoyin	Hand jueyin

(Continued)

125

Radial Pulse Positions and Correspondences *(Continued)*			
After Wang Shuhe (Mai Jing, circa 280 A.D.)			
Pulse Position	**Depth**	**Left Side**	**Right Side**
Inch (Distal)	*Superficial*	Small Intestine	Large Intestine
	Deep	Heart	Lung
Barrier (Middle)	*Superficial*	Gallbladder	Spleen
	Deep	Liver	Stomach
Foot (Proximal)	*Superficial*	Bladder	Triple Burner
	Deep	Kidney	Mingmen
After Li Shizhen (Bin Hu Mo Xue, 1564 A.D.)			
Radial Position		**Left Side**	**Right Side**
Inch (Distal)		Heart	Lungs
Barrier (Middle)		Liver/Gallbladder	Spleen/Stomach
Foot (Proximal)		Kidney, Small Intestine, Bladder	Mingmen
After Zhang Jiebin (Jing Yue Quan Shu, 1624 A.D.)			
Inch (Distal)	*Superficial*	Heart Governor	Sternum
	Deep	Heart	Lungs
Barrier (Middle)	*Superficial*	Gallbladder	Stomach
	Deep	Liver	Spleen
Foot (Proximal)	*Superficial*	BL, LI	TB, SI, Mingmen
	Deep	Left Kidney	Right Kidney

15.2 Radial Pulses and Their Clinical Significance

Radial Pulses and Their Clinical Significance		
Pulse	**Characteristics**	**Clinical Significance**
Floating	Superabundant at the superficial level and insufficient at the deep level	Exterior exogenous contraction pattern. A floating pulse in an enduring disease or during hemorrhage is a negative sign
Deep	Not felt until heavy pressure is applied	Interior pattern
Slow	3 beats or less per respiration	Cold pattern, yang depletion
Rapid	6 beats or more per respiration	Heat pattern or yin depletion
Depleted	Very weak and relatively small; a general term for all forceless pulses	Depletion, especially of yang
Replete	Very strong and relatively large. A general term for all forceful pulses.	Repletion patterns
Slippery	Rises and falls smoothly, like pearls rolling in a dish	Pregnancy, phlegm patterns, digestate accumulation
Rough	Relatively weak; rises disfluently, like a knife scraping bamboo	Blood depletion or stasis
Wiry	Usually forceful; long and straight, like a guitar string	Hepatocystic disease, phlegm-rheum, pain
Soggy	Relatively weak; slightly floating and fine. Also called a soft pulse	Depletion of blood and qi, damp encumbrance
Surging	Strong; broad and large, falls away weakly after an exuberant onset	Heat, pathogen exuberance, depletion fire

(Continued)

Radial Pulses and Their Clinical Significance
(Continued)

Pulse	Characteristics	Clinical Significance
Faint	Very weak; fine, faint, and indistinct, sometimes felt and sometimes not	Depletion desertion of qi and blood
Fine	Generally very weak; thin and threadlike. Also called a small pulse	Insufficiency of qi and blood, and especially of qi and yin
Weak	Deep and forceless; fine and small	Insufficiency of blood and qi
Large	Broad and large; refers to pulse size, no connotation of strength	Pathogen exuberance, advancing condition, underlying depletion.
Scattered	Very weak; floating and forceless, large and without root	Dissipation of qi and blood, impending expiry of essential qi
Tight	Strong; wiry and markedly forceful	Cold and pain
Scallion Stalk	Weak (forceless when heavy pressure is applied); floating and empty in the middle, like a scallion stalk	Blood collapse, seminal loss; commonly occurs in massive bleeding
Drumskin	Weak (forceless when heavy pressure is applied), occurring with wiry pulse	Blood collapse, seminal loss, commonly occurs in massive bleeding
Confined	Deep and forceful	Cold pain, inner body exuberance of yin cold; commonly referred to as a deep wiry pulse or a deep replete pulse

(Continued)

Radial Pulses and Their Clinical Significance *(Continued)*		
Pulse	**Characteristics**	**Clinical Significance**
Racing	7 or more beats per respiration	Basically the same as a rapid pulse, but suggests depletion
Animated	6 or more beats per respiration; soft, slippery, rapid, bouncing like beans	High fever, palpitations, pregnancy
Hidden	Deeper than a deep pulse	Inner body pathogen block, fulminant desertion of yang qi
Moderate	3 - 4 beats per respiration	Normal
Rapid irregularly interrupted	6 or more beats per respiration, pausing irregularly	Debilitation of organ qi, obstruction of heart blood or heart qi flow; sometimes seen in healthy persons
Slow irregularly interrupted	4 or less beats per respiration, pausing irregularly	Debilitation of organ qi, obstruction of heart blood or heart qi flow. Sometimes seen in healthy persons
Regularly interrupted	Relatively regular pauses	Organ qi debilitation; impact trauma
Long	Extending beyond barrier and cubit positions	Counterflow qi, fire exuberance, other surfeit patterns
Short	Felt only at barrier	Qi and blood depletion, as well as other insufficiency patterns

Yin and Yang Pulses

Yin Pulses

Sunken (deep)	Internal obstruction
Slow	Cold pathogen
Thin	Depleted blood or qi
Empty	Depleted blood and qi
Knotted (slow, irregular)	Cold obstructs qi or blood
Short	General depletion
Choppy (uneven, rough)	Depleted blood or essence if thin; or congealed blood
Regularly intermittent	Serious heart problem, organs exhausted
Hidden	*If strong:* cold obstructing channels *If weak:* depleted yang
Hollow (scallion stalk)	Depleted blood

Yang Pulses

Floating, superficial	If forceful: exogenous pathogen If without strength: depleted yin
Rapid	Heat pathogen
Large	Repletion; heat in stomach or intestines
Replete	Repletion of qi or blood
Hurried (rapid, irregular)	Heat pathogen agitates qi and blood
Long	General repletion
Slippery	Damp, mucus; sign of pregnancy
Wiry	Liver or gallbladder problem, endogenous wind
Tight	Repletion, cold, stagnation

15.3 *Nei Jing* Pulse Diagnosis

According to the *Nei Jing* (Su Wen, ch. 20), the body is divided into three sections, Heaven (upper), Human (central), and Earth (lower), each of which has three locations, also referred to as Heaven, Human, and Earth. These sectional divisions were located over major arteries, the palpation of which was used to determine the state of qi and blood in their respective areas, as described in the following table. Although no specific acupoints were named, they can be deduced from the text. Where disagreement exists, alternate positions have been indicated in brackets.

The Nine Pulse Locations in the Three Body Sections			
Body	**Relative Position**	**Location of Pulse**	**Measures**
Heaven [upper body]	Heaven	GB-3 [GB-4, GB-7]	Qi of temporal area
	Human	TB-21 [TB-22]	Qi of eyes and ears
	Earth	ST-3 [ST-6, ST-9]	Qi of mouth and teeth
Human [middle body]	Heaven	LU-9	Lung qi
	Human	HT-7	Heart qi
	Earth	LI-4 [LI-3]	Thoracic [*tanzhong*] qi
Earth [lower body]	Heaven	LV-10 [LV-3]	Liver qi
	Human	SP-11 [ST-42]	Spleen and stomach qi
	Earth	KI-3	Kidney qi

15.4 *Shanghan Lun* Pulse Diagnosis

The *Shanghan Lun* simplified the above method, using one position each in the upper, middle, and lower sections of the body. This method has proven useful in clinical practice and is still employed by many practitioners.

Shanghan Lun Pulse Diagnosis		
Body Section	**Location of Pulse**	**Measures**
Upper body	ST-9	Measures general state of yang, ascent of qi, quantity and quality of qi in upper body
Lower body	ST-42	Measures general state of yin, descent of qi, quantity and quality of qi in lower body
Middle body	*Cunkou*	Gauges qi in twelve channels (it is unclear whether this refers to LU-9, or the radial pulses as a whole)
Note: KI-3 is usually added to the above to gauge the state of *yuan* (original) qi.		

15.5 Palpation of Channels and Points

Palpation of Channels and Points	
Characteristics	**Indications**
Tenderness at Alarm-mu points; tension or nodules at back transport-shu points	Disorder of associated organs
Tenderness at ST-36	Gastralgia, duodenal ulcer
Tenderness at lanwei (M-LE-13)	Appendicitis
Tenderness at dannang (M-LE-23)	Gallbladder disorders

15.6 Abdominal Palpation

The emphasis in this chapter on radial pulse palpation, rather than palpation of the abdomen or of the channels, reflects common practice. However, though abdominal diagnosis has not yet achieved a prominent place in the mainstream of American acupuncture practice, it is an extremely valuable approach to confirming illness patterns and structuring treatment strategies. The reader is urged to refer to Matsumoto and Birch, *Hara Diagnosis: Reflections on the Sea*, for an in-depth presentation of the subject. In particular, see chapter 2 for an introduction to palpation, and pp. 259-262 for a detailed presentation of common patterns of abdominal reactivity.

Abdominal Palpation	
Characteristics	**Indications**
Distention with tympanic note on percussion, but normal urination	Qi stagnation
Distention with gurgling sound on palpation, fluctuating sensation	Fluid accumulation
Immovable, hard masses	Static blood
Unfixed, soft masses	Stagnant qi
Masses clustered in lower left quadrant, with constipation	Retention of dry stool
Rebounding pain in right lower quadrant	Qi and blood stasis, appendicitis

Abdominal Differential Diagnosis *(After Matsumoto and Birch)*	
Reactive Region	**General Indications**
Subcostal, bilateral	Yinwei mai—chong mai, liver (possibly spleen) depletion
Subcostal, right side	Liver problems, yinwei mai—chong mai, "Cross Syndrome"
Subcostal, left side	Spleen depletion, yinwei mai—chong mai
Substernal	Heart problem, yinwei mai—chong mai

Continued

Abdominal Differential Diagnosis *(Continued)*	
Reactive Region	**General Indications**
Supra-umbilical midline	Spleen depletion, spleen-stomach problems, yinqiao mai—ren mai
Periumbilical	Spleen depletion, spleen-stomach problems, yinqiao mai—ren mai, yinwei mai—chong mai, yangwei mai—dai mai
Sub-umbilical	Kidney depletion, yinqiao mai—ren mai
Left of umbilicus	Liver problems, intestinal problems
Right of umbilicus	Lung depletion, intestinal problems liver problems
Anterior superior iliac spine	Gallbladder channel, yangwei mai—dai mai, yangqiao mai—du mai, yinqiao mai—ren mai, "Cross" syndrome
KI-16	Spleen depletion, kidney depletion, kidney channel problems, chong mai—Yinwei mai, yinqiao mai—ren mai, daimai—yangwei mai
ST-25	Liver problems, lung depletion (when reactivity is on right ST-25), triple burner channel problems
LV-14	Liver depletion, liver channel problems, yinwei mai—chong mai, "Cross Syndrome"
LU-1	Lung depletion, lung channel problems, ren mai—yinqiao mai
CV-12	Spleen depletion, spleen-stomach problems, renmai—yinqiao mai
CV-6	Kidney depletion, ren mai—yinqiao mai

Part VI

Strategies
for
Point Selection

16 Five-Phase Treatment

16.1 Commonly Used Chinese Five-Phase Point Combinations

16.1.1 Matching

To prevent a repletion illness from changing and spreading, first supplement that phase which could be affected (i.e., the "conquered" or "grandchild" phase, according to the control cycle), using its own "phase" point and its "mother" point on its associated channel. Then, drain the originally affected channel, using its own phase point and its "child" point.

Example: Diagnosis reveals liver (wood) repletion; according to the control cycle, this repletion should normally transmit its illness to the spleen (earth). So, first supplement the earth point of earth, SP-3, and next supplement the mother (fire) point of earth, SP-2. Then, drain the wood point of wood, LV-1, and finally drain its child (fire) point, LV-2.

16.1.2 Mother-Child

When both mother and child phases are replete, reduce the mother channel only, using its own phase point and its child point. Likewise, if both mother and child phases are both depleted, supplement the child channel only, using its own phase point and its mother point (cf. *Nanjing*, ch. 75: "The child can make its mother replete; the mother can make her child depleted.").

16.1.3 Brother-Sister

When coupled yin-yang channels are *both* affected, in cases of repletion drain the phase point and the child point on each channel, and in cases of depletion supplement the phase point and the mother point of each channel.

Example: For concurrent hyperactivity of liver and gallbladder, drain wood and fire on the liver channel, LV-1 and LV-2, along with draining wood and fire on the gallbladder channel, GB-41 and GB-38.

16.1.4 Uprooting the Source

After needling other appropriate points on a channel, needle the source point. If depleted, supplement; if replete, drain.

Example: To supplement the liver channel, first supplement its "mother" point, LV-8, and then supplement its source point, LV-3. When draining the liver channel, first drain the "child" point, LV-2, and then drain the source point, LV-3.

16.2 Treatment by the Mother-Child Rule

According to five-phase theory, when a particular phase is depleted, the phase preceding it in the engendering cycle (the "mother" phase) must be supplemented. Likewise, when a particular phase is replete, the phase following it in the engendering cycle (the "child") phase, must be drained.

Each of the five transporting-*shu* points has a five-phase correspondence; also, each of the twelve primary channels, via its related organ, has its own five-phase correspondence. There are, therefore, two ways to apply the above rule. First, a point on the channel associated with the affected phase may be chosen: e.g., if the lung — associated with metal — is depleted, LU-9, the earth point on the lung channel (earth is the "mother" of metal) may be supplemented. Second, the "mother" phase point on the "mother" phase channel may be supplemented: in this example, SP-3, the earth point of the earth channel, would be used. If a particular phase was in a state of repletion, the principle is the same: drain the "child" point on the affected channel, and additionally drain the "child" point on the channel associated with the "child" phase.

The "mother" or "child" *channel* referred to in the following table is *not* the channel preceding or succeeding the affected channel in the superficial ("Chinese clock") circulation of qi. Rather, it is the channel associated with the *zang-fu* organ system of the preceding or succeeding phase (refer to the illustration of the five-phase cycles on page 20).

Use of Transporting-*shu* Points			
Channel Condition		Treatment via Affected Channel	Treatment via Mother or Child Channel
Lung	Depletion	LU-9, earth of metal channel	SP-3, earth of earth channel
	Repletion	LU-5, water of metal channel	KI-10, water of water channel
Heart	Depletion	HT-9, wood of fire channel	LV-1, wood of wood channel
	Repletion	HT-7, earth of fire channel	SP-3, earth of earth channel
Pericard-ium	Depletion	PC-9, wood of fire channel	LV-1, wood of wood channel
	Repletion	PC-7, earth of fire channel	SP-3, earth of earth channel
Large Intestine	Depletion	LI-11, earth of metal channel	ST-36, earth of earth channel
	Repletion	LI-2, water of metal channel	BL-66, water of water channel

(Continued)

Use of Transporting-*shu* Points *(Continued)*			
Channel Condition		**Treatment via Affected Channel**	**Treatment via Mother or Child Channel**
Small Intestine	Depletion	SI-3, wood of fire channel	GB-41, wood of wood channel
	Repletion	SI-8, earth of fire channel	ST-36, earth of earth channel
Triple Burner	Depletion	TB-3, wood of fire channel	GB-41, wood of wood channel
	Repletion	TB-10, earth of fire channel	ST-36, earth of earth channel
Spleen	Depletion	SP-2, fire of earth channel	HT-8, fire of fire channel
	Repletion	SP-5, metal of earth channel	LU-8, metal of metal channel
Kidney	Depletion	KI-7, metal of water channel	LU-8, metal of metal channel
	Repletion	KI-1, wood of water channel	LV-I, wood of wood channel
Liver	Depletion	LV-8 water of wood channel	KI-10, water of water channel
	Repletion	LV-2, fire of wood channel	HT-8, fire of fire channel
Stomach	Depletion	ST-41, fire of earth channel	SI-5, fire of fire channel
	Repletion	ST-45, metal of earth channel	LU-1, metal of metal channel
Bladder	Depletion	BL-67, metal of water channel	LI-1, metal of metal channel
	Repletion	BL-65, wood of water channel	GB-41, wood of wood channel
Gall-bladder	Depletion	GB-43, water of wood channel	BL-66, water of water channel
	Repletion	GB-38, fire of wood channel	SI-5, fire of fire channel

16.3 Korean Four-Point Five-Phase Treatment

In the sixteenth century, the Korean Buddhist monk Sa-Am extended the above theory even further. He felt that treatments could be made more effective by not only supplementing the mother phase in cases of depletion, but by additionally draining the controlling phase on the same and the related channel. To cite the example in the above section (lung-metal depletion), not only would LU-9 (earth of metal) and SP-3 (earth of earth) be supplemented, but additionally, LU-10 (fire of metal) and HT-8 (fire of fire — some sources prefer PC-8, considering heart fire as sacred and not to be used), would be drained.

Conversely, if the lungs were overactive (replete), LU-5 (water of metal) plus KI-10 (water of water) would be drained, while LU-10 (fire of metal) and HT-8 or PC-8 (fire of fire) would be supplemented.

Stated simply, in this example, for lung, i.e., metal, depletion: a) supplement earth of metal plus earth of earth; b) drain fire of metal plus fire of fire. For lung-metal repletion: a) drain water of metal plus water of water; b) supplement fire of metal plus fire of fire.

This method may also be used to treat cold and heat illnesses. Instead of using supplementation and drainage points, use fire and water points on the affected channels, as shown in the tables which follow.

There are several methods to implement this technique. Many Korean practitioners use a spring-loaded "flying needle" technique, rapidly supplementing or draining points according to direction of channel flow. Other practitioners use more traditional supplementation and draining techniques, e.g., in cases of depletion, first inserting needles at the supplementing points, and removing them before inserting needles at the draining points. The reverse would hold in cases of repletion. Other practitioners have used gold and silver needles, simultaneously inserted, to good effect.

Korean four-point technique is the foundation for modern Korean constitutional acupuncture. A detailed discussion of this sophisticated system is outside the scope of this text.

Korean Four-Point Five-Phase Treatments
Depletion and Repletion Patterns

Channel	Depletion Patterns				Repletion Patterns			
	Supplement		Drain		Supplement		Drain	
LU	SP-3	LU-9	HT-8	LU-10	HT-8	LU-10	KI-10	LU-5
LI	ST-36	LI-11	SI-5	LI-5	SI-5	LI-5	BL-66	LI-2
ST	SI-5	ST-41	GB-41	ST-43	GB-41	ST-43	LI-1	ST-45
SP	HT-8	SP-2	LV-1	SP-1	LV-1	SP-1	LU-8	SP-5
HT	LV-1	HT-9	KI-10	HT-3	KI-10	HT-3	SP-3	HT-7
SI	GB-41	SI-3	BL-66	SI-2	BL-66	SI-2	ST-36	SI-8
BL	LI-1	BL-67	ST-36	BL-54	ST-36	BL-54	GB-41	BL-65
KI	LU-8	KI-7	SP-3	KI-3	SP-3	KI-3	LV-1	KI-1
PC	LV-1	PC-9	KI-10	PC-3	KI-10	PC-3	SP-3	PC-7
TW	GB-41	TW-3	BL-66	TW-2	BL-66	TW-2	ST-36	TW-10
GB	BL-66	GB-43	LI-1	GB-44	LI-1	GB-44	SI-5	GB-38
LV	KI-10	LV-8	LU-8	LV-4	LU-8	LV-4	HT-8	LV-2

Korean Four-Point Five-Phase Treatments								
Cold and Heat Patterns								
Channel	Cold Patterns				Heat Patterns			
	Supplement		Drain		Supplement		Drain	
LU	HT-8	LU-10	LU-5	KI-10	LU-5	KI-10	SP-3	LU-9
LI	SI-5	ST-41	BL-66	LI-2	LI-2	BL-66	SI-5	ST-41
ST	ST-41	SI-5	ST-44	BL-66	ST-44	BL-66	ST-36	BL-54
SP	SP-2	HT-8	SP-9	KI-10	SP-9	KI-10	SP-3	KI-3
HT	HT-8	KI-2	HT-3	KI-10	HT-3	KI-10	HT-8	KI-2
SI	SI-5	BL-60	SI-2	BL-66	SI-2	BL-66	SI-8	ST-36
BL	SI-5	BL-60	SI-2	BL-66	SI-2	BL-66	ST-36	BL-54
KI	HT-8	KI-2	KI-10	HT-3	KI-10	HT-3	SP-3	KI-3
PC	HT-8	PC-8	PC-3	HT-3	PC-3	HT-3	SP-3	PC-7
TW	TW-6	BL-60	TW-2	BL-66	TW-2	BL-66	TW-6	BL-60
GB	GB-38	SI-5	GB-43	BL-66	GB-43	BL-66	BL-54	GB-34
LV	LV-2	HT-8	KI-10	LV-8	KI-10	LV-8	LV-3	SP-3

16.4 Chinese Six-Point Five-Phase Treatments

According to five phase theory, whenever one phase is affected, two related phases are secondarily affected. Six-point treatment takes the Korean method described above one step farther by utilizing not only the points and channels of the phase that *controls* the primarily affected phase, but also those of the phase *controlled by* the primarily affected phase. For example, in a case of liver (wood) depletion:

Step One: Supplement the water point of the wood channel (LV-8) plus the water point of the water channel (KI-10);

Step Two: Drain the metal point of the wood channel (LV-4) plus the metal point of the metal channel (LU-8);

Step Three: Furthermore, drain the earth point of the wood channel (LV-3) plus the earth point of the earth channel (SP-3).

Cases of repletion follow the same principle, draining the primarily affected phase, then supplementing both the phase controlling and the phase controlled by the primarily affected phase.

Chinese Six-Point Five Phase Treatments *Depletion Patterns*							
Depleted Phase		**Supplement**		*Drain*			
Wood		**Water**		*Metal*		*Earth*	
	LV	**LV-8**	**KI-10**	*LV-4*	*LU-8*	*LV-3*	*SP-3*
	GB	**GB-43**	**BL-66**	*GB-44*	*LI-1*	*GB-34*	*ST-36*
Fire		**Wood**		*Water*		*Metal*	
	HT	**HT-9**	**LV-1**	*HT-3*	*KI-10*	*HT-4*	*LU-8*
	SI	**SI-3**	**GB-41**	*SI-2*	*BL-66*	*SI-1*	*LI-1*
Earth		**Fire**		*Wood*		*Water*	
	SP	**SP-2**	**HT-8**	*SP-1*	*LV-1*	*SP-9*	*KI-10*
	ST	**ST-41**	**SI-5**	*ST-43*	*GB-41*	*ST-44*	*BL-66*
Metal		**Earth**		*Fire*		*Wood*	
	LU	**LU-9**	**SP-3**	*LU-10*	*HT-8*	*LU-11*	*LV-1*
	LI	**LI-11**	**ST-36**	*LI-5*	*SI-5*	*LI-3*	*GB-41*
Water		**Metal**		*Earth*		*Fire*	
	KI	**KI-7**	**LU-8**	*KI-3*	*SP-3*	*KI-2*	*HT-8*
	BL	**BL-67**	**LI-1**	*BL-40*	*ST-36*	*BL-60*	*SI-5*
Fire (Ministerial)		**Wood**		*Water*		*Metal*	
	PC	**PC-9**	**LV-1**	*PC-3*	*KI-10*	*PC-5*	*LU-8*
	TB	**TB-3**	**GB-41**	*TB-2*	*BL-66*	*TB-1*	*ST-45*

Chinese Six-Point Five Phase Treatments *Repletion Patterns*							
Replete *Phase*		*Drain*		**Supplement**			
Wood		*Fire*		**Metal**		**Earth**	
	LV	*LV-2*	*HT-8*	**LV-4**	**LU-8**	**LV-3**	**SP-3**
	GB	*GB-38*	*SI-5*	**GB-44**	**LI-1**	**GB-34**	**ST-36**
Fire		*Earth*		**Water**		**Metal**	
	HT	*HT-7*	*SP-3*	**HT-3**	**KI-10**	**HT-4**	**LU-8**
	SI	*SI-8*	*ST-36*	**SI-2**	**BL-66**	**SI-1**	**LI-1**
Earth		*Metal*		**Wood**		**Water**	
	SP	*SP-5*	*LU-8*	**SP-1**	**LV-1**	**SP-9**	**KI-10**
	ST	*ST-45*	*LI-1*	**ST-43**	**GB-41**	**ST-44**	**BL-66**
Metal		*Water*		**Fire**		**Wood**	
	LU	*LU-5*	*KI-10*	**LU-10**	**HT-8**	**LU-11**	**LV-1**
	LI	*LI-2*	*BL-66*	**LI-5**	**SI-5**	**LI-3**	**GB-41**
Water		*Wood*		**Earth**		**Fire**	
	KI	*KI-1*	*LV-1*	**KI-3**	**SP-3**	**KI-2**	**HT-8**
	BL	*BL-65*	*GB-41*	**BL-40**	**ST-36**	**BL-60**	**SI-5**
Fire (Ministerial)		*Earth*		**Water**		**Metal**	
	PC	*PC-7*	*SP-3*	**PC-3**	**KI-10**	**PC-5**	**LU-8**
	TB	*TB-10*	*ST-36*	**TB-2**	**BL-66**	**TB-1**	**ST-45**

(From *Zhenjiu Wushuxue Yingyung*, pp. 57, 59).

16.5 *Nan Jing* Five-Phase Point Selection

16.5.1 Point Selection According to the Traditional Functions of the Transporting-*shu* Points

Western acupuncture literature has all but ignored the so-called "traditional functions" of the five transporting-*shu* points, as outlined in *Nan Jing* ch. 68   see section **8.1**. Actually, these constitute the basis for a rather sophisticated method of point selection based on systematic diagnostic criteria. Each point function typifies a *general category* of symptoms, which will be found to relate to that point's associated phase and organ function.

Five Transporting-*shu* Points: Traditional Applications				
Point	Phase	Organ	Traditional Applications	General Symptoms
Well-jing	Wood	LV/GB	Fullness below the heart	Any pathogenic stagnation
Spring-ying	Fire	HT/SI	Heat, fever	Any febrile or inflammatory condition
Stream-shu	Earth	SP/ST	Heavy limbs, arthralgia	Any rheumatic, damp, or *bi* pattern
River-jing	Metal	LU/LI	Coughing, dyspnea	Respiratory problems, asthma, etc.
Uniting-he	Water	KI/BL	Qi reversals, diarrhea	Counterflow qi patterns, excretory disturbances

Later commentators, including Lu Guang (third century), Wang Haogu (thirteenth century), and Hua Shou (fourteenth century), deduced the following method: when the pulse of a certain *zang* or *fu* organ was accompanied by certain diagnostic "confirmations," and furthermore was accompanied by symptoms belonging to one of the above categories, the corresponding point on that organ's particular channel would be chosen. "Exterior confirmations" implied that the *fu* organ aspect of that phase was affected, while "interior confirmations" implicated the *zang* organ.

For example: If the patient is found to have a wiry pulse, i.e., one corresponding to wood, with interior confirmations such as urinary drip, difficult defecation, muscle spasms, etc., together with fullness below the heart or some other pathologic stagnation, then LV-1, the well-*jing* point of the liver channel would be chosen. If the patient has *exterior* symptoms such as fastidiousness, a cyan complexion, and irritability, plus fullness below the heart, etc., then GB-44, the well-*jing* point of the gallbladder channel, would be used.

Nan Jing Five-Phase Point Selection
External and Internal Confirmation

Affected Organ	Associated Pulse	Confirmation	
Gallbladder	Wiry	External	Fastidiousness; short temper; cyan complexion
Liver		Internal	Heavy, painful limbs with difficulty walking; urinary drip; constipation; cramps; pulse or accumulation to the left of the navel
Small Intestine	Floating and Surging	External	Reddish complexion; dry mouth; frequent laughter
Heart		Internal	Restlessness; oppressive feeling in the chest; heart pains; hot palms; dry heaves; pulse or accumulation above navel
Stomach	Floating and moderate	External	Yellowish complexion; belching; preoccupation; desire for tasty food
Spleen		Internal	Abdominal distention and fullness; food not digested; body feels heavy; joint pains; weariness; desire to lie down; inability to bend limbs; pulse directly at naval
Large Intestine	Floating	External	White complexion (pallor); sneezing; frequent tearfulness; melancholy; grief
Lung		Internal	Dyspnea; cough; shivering from chills and fever; pulse at right side of naval
Bladder	Deep and Slow	External	Blackish complexion; frequent yawning; fearfulness
Kidney		Internal	Qi ascending counterflow; acute lower abdominal pain; diarrhea with heavy, sinking sensation; cold and counterflow in feet and calves; pulse below the naval

Note: The pulses referred to here are general pulse qualities, as opposed to the pulse of a particular organ. Also, note that the traditional differentiation of phase association between the *zang* and *fu* channels is not taken into account in this system.

Nan Jing Five-Phase Point Selection *Associated Symptoms and Point Selection*					
Affected Organ	**Associated Symptoms and Point Selection**				
	Fullness below heart *(Well-jing)*	Body heat *(Spring-ying)*	Heavy body, joint pain *(Stream-shu)*	Dyspnea, cough chills & fever *(River-jing)*	Counterflow Qi *(Uniting-he)*
Gallbladder	GB-44	GB-43	GB-41	GB-38	GB-34
Liver	LV-1	LV-2	LV-3	LV-4	LV-8
Small Intestine	SI-1	SI-2	SI-3	SI-5	SI-8
Heart	HT-9	HT-8	HT-7	HT-4	HT-3
Stomach	ST-45	ST-44	ST-43	ST-41	ST-36
Spleen	SP-1	SP-2	SP-3	SP-5	SP-9
Large Intestine	LI-1	LI-2	LI-3	LI-5	LI-11
Lung	LU-11	LU-10	LU-9	LU-8	LU-5
Bladder	BL-67	BL-66	BL-65	BL-60	BL-40
Kidney	KI-1	KI-2	KI-3	KI-7	KI-10

(From *Zhenjiu Wushuxue Yingyung*, pp. 42-46).

For a more thorough understanding of the principles underlying this method, compare chapters 16, 68, and 74 in Unschuld's *Nan Ching*.

16.5.2 North-South Five-Phase Point Selection

Nan Jing, ch. 75 states: "When the east is replete and the west is depleted, drain the south and supplement the north." This is an example of "using what is not yet ill to treat what is already ill." For a more complete explanation of the rather complex rationale behind this treatment strategy, see Unschuld's *Nan Ching*, ch. 75.

North-South Point Selection				
Disease Pattern	Distinguishing Characteristics	Treatment Principle	Points Selected	
			Yin Channels	Yang Channels
Liver repletion with Lung depletion	Spleen (earth) remains unaffected	Supplement water on water channels	KI-10 KI-7	BL-66 BL-67
		Drain fire on fire channels	HT-8 HT-7	SI-5 SI-8
Heart repletion with Kidney depletion	Lung (metal) remains unaffected	Supplement wood on wood channels	LV-1 LV-8	GB-41 GB-43
		Drain earth on earth channels	SP-3 SP-5	ST-36 ST-45
Spleen repletion with Liver depletion	Kidney (water) remains unaffected	Supplement fire on fire channels	HT-8 HT-9	SI-5 SI-3
		Drain metal on metal channels	LU-8 LU-5	LI-1 LI-2
Liver repletion with Heart depletion	Liver (wood) remains unaffected	Supplement earth on earth channels	SP-3 SP-2	ST-36 ST-41
		Drain water on water channels	KI-10 KI-1	BL-66 BL-65
Kidney repletion with Spleen depletion	Heart (fire) remains unaffected	Supplement metal on metal channels	LU-8 LU-9	LI-1 LI-11
		Drain wood on wood channels	LV-1 LV-2	GB-41 GB-38

Note: The *Nan Jing* does not specify which points to use for draining and supplementation. Some commentators suggest the phase point itself, while others suggest the mother or child points. Presumably, one could be used to supplement the effects of the other. Both are included here for reference.

16.6 Five-Phase Qi-Transfer Theory and its Application

This method of balancing replete (excessive) and depleted (deficient) organs is based on the notion that qi may be transferred from one organ to another via the five phase-related (or "elemental") points on each channel. Although rarely mentioned in modern Chinese texts, it is popular among European practitioners, and among graduates of the schools founded by the British acupuncturist J.R. Worsley. It may also be found in certain Korean and Japanese traditions as well.

Either the *sheng* (engendering) or *ke* (restraining) cycles may be used to determine point selection. The cycle chosen is usually the one which allows the shortest route from imbalanced to balanced organ. Supplementation (tonification) should always precede draining (dispersion); thus, the depleted organ is always acted upon first. If an imbalance exists between a yin *zang* organ and a yang *fu* organ — or vice versa — the *luo* point of one of the channels may be used as well. Repletion or depletion is determined entirely from the pulses. Successful treatment is determined by a qualitative change in pulse amplitude and force. Three illustrative examples follow:

Example 1: The large intestine pulse is weak, while the stomach pulse is quite strong, showing depletion and repletion in their respective organs. In five-phase terms, yang metal is weak and yang earth is too strong. The repletion in earth must therefore be shifted to metal, which is done by simply stimulating the earth point on the metal channel, LI-11.

Example 2: The pulses show an excess in the liver, and a depletion in the stomach. The spleen pulse is normal. Here, the imbalance exists between a yin and yang organ. First, transfer energy from the normal yin spleen-earth to the depleted yang stomach-earth through the *luo* point of the stomach, ST-40. Then, using the *ke* cycle, drain the excess of yin liver-wood to yin spleen-earth by stimulating the wood point of yin earth, SP-1.

Example 3: The liver pulse is full and replete, while the lung pulse is empty and depleted. Normally, metal should control wood, and energy cannot be transferred counterflow along either the engendering or control cycles. Consequently, the depleted lung-metal must first be supplemented by transferring energy from spleen-earth via the normal *sheng* cycle, using the earth point of metal, LU-9. Then, the replete liver-wood energy may be drained into spleen-earth across the normal *ke* cycle, using the wood point of earth, SP-1.

The last treatment could also be done simply by using the *sheng* cycle. First, bring energy from spleen-earth to lung-metal by stimulating the earth point of metal, LU-9; then, move energy from pericardium-fire (the heart-fire channel is usually avoided) to spleen-earth by stimulating the fire point of earth, SP-2. Finally, drain the replete energy of liver-wood into pericardium-fire through the wood point of ministerial fire, PC-9.

17 Eight Method Acupuncture

<table>
<tr><th colspan="3">Eight Method Acupuncture</th></tr>
<tr><th>Method</th><th>Neijing Reference</th><th>Treatment</th></tr>
<tr>
<td>*Diaphoresis*</td>
<td>"If the illness is in the skin, use diaphoresis to diffuse it." (*SW* V, 4:4)

"If the body is as hot as burning coals, use diaphoresis and it will dissipate." (*SW* III, 2:1)</td>
<td>Vigorously drain **LI-4** until profuse sweating occurs. If the sweating does not stop, needle **ST-33** and supplement **LI-4**.</td>
</tr>
<tr>
<td>*Emesis*</td>
<td>"If (the illness) is in the upper regions, make it pass up and out." (*SW* V, 4:4)</td>
<td>Vigorously needle **PC-6** countercurrent until the patient vomits. If the vomit does not cease, supplement **ST-36**.</td>
</tr>
<tr>
<td>*Precipitation (Purgation)*</td>
<td>"If the center is full, drain it via the inner (passages)." (*SW* V, 4:4)</td>
<td>Drain **SP-6**. If the purgation is too profuse, supplement **LI-4**. In heat illnesses add **ST-25**, **CV-6**, and **ST-36**.</td>
</tr>
<tr>
<td>*Harmonization*</td>
<td>"The method of harmonization requires making yin and yang communicate." (*LS* IX, 1)</td>
<td>Regulate the stomach through **ST-36**; course qi through **LV-3**; open depression (of liver qi, etc.) with **PC-6**.</td>
</tr>
<tr>
<td>*Warming*</td>
<td>"If the (bodily) form is insufficient, warm it through the qi." (*SW* V, 4:4)

"If there is cold, heat it; if there is coolness, warm it." (*SW* LXXIV, 2:5)</td>
<td>Supplement and warm **CV-12**, **CV-8**, **CV-6**, **ST-36**, and **GV-4**.</td>
</tr>
<tr>
<td>*Cooling*</td>
<td>"If there is warmth, cool it." (*SW* XX, 2)</td>
<td>Drain **LV-2**, **LI-11**, **BL-40**, **LU-5**, **GB-20**. For extreme heat, bleed the 12 well-*jing* points.</td>
</tr>
</table>

(Continued)

Eight Method Acupuncture		
(Continued)		
Method	**Neijing Reference**	**Treatment**
Supplementing (Tonifying)	"Supplement depletion." (*SW XX, 2*)	Supplement and/or moxa **GV-14, GV-12, GV-4, BL-23, CV-4, CV-6, CV-12, ST-36.**
Draining (Sedating)	"Drain repletions." (*SW XX, 2*) "Pare away firmness." (*SW LXXIV, 5:2*) "If there is repletion, dissipate and drain it." (*SW V. 4:4*) "If there is old stagnation, eliminate it." (*SW LV, 1*).	If the eyes are inflamed, drain **M-HN-9** (*taiyang*) and **GB-20**; for abdominal distention and bloating, drain **CV-12, LV-13, CV-9**; for wind pathogen repletion, drain **CV-22 and ST-40**, retaining the needle for some time.

(From *Zhenjiu Linchuang Shouci*, pp. 80,81).

18 Common Point Combinations for Specific Treatment Objectives

Theories of point selection often develop in the wake of clinical experience, justifying theoretically what physicians already know to be true through clinical trial. Strategy in this sense is largely dependent on familiarization with a finite set of point groups: in a word, formulae.

The following list presents some 300 common point combinations for specific treatment applications, derived from common treatments for specific disorders. It is meant to provide a self-study tool for review of commonly accepted treatment methods and point combinations: in no way should it be considered exhaustive.

For clarity of presentation, we have departed from the boxed-table format in presenting these point combinations. Daggers (†) after point entries indicate that application of moxa is appropriate.

Activate blood to promote menstrual flow..SP-10
Aphonia, relieve..HT-5, CV-23
Appendicitis, empirical point for..M-LE-13 (*lanwei*)

Bladder channel pain, course..BL-40 (bleed), BL-58
Bladder function, regulate..BL-28, CV-3
Bladder qi, supplement..BL-28†, CV-3†
Bladder, regulate to promote urination CV-3
Blood flow, invigorate and stop pain SP-8, SP-10
Blood heat, cool LI-11, SP-10
Blood heat, eliminate ....SP-10, BL-40 (bleed)
Blood production, fortify...BL-20, BL-21, ST-36
Blood, cool PC-3
Blood, nourish and calm the spirit..SP-6, BL-20, HT-7
Blood, regulate PC-6, SP-4
Blood, supplement BL-18, BL-20, ST-36
Blood, supplement by boosting qi CV-12, ST-36, SP-6
Bones, strengthen to relieve lumbar and knee pain M-BW-24
Breast, ease pain and distention in GB-41

Central fullness, relieve CV-12, ST-36
Channels, clear heat from GV-14
Channels, clear...LI-4, LV-3
Chest and diaphragm, ease CV-14, BL-17
Chest, relieve depression and fullness in, regulate upper burner qi PC-6
Chest, relieve pressure in CV-17
Chills and fever, reduce..LI-4, TB-5
Circulation of qi and blood, normalize to clear channels LI-4, LV-3
Circulation, activate in taiyang and GV to expel pathogen SI-3, BL-12
Cold, internal, dispel...CV-6 (ginger moxa)

CV yin motility, open to activate kidney and move water LU-7, KI-6
Conception and penetrating vessels, regulate.................................CV-7†
Consciousness, restore GV-26
Constipation, fluid depletion type, relieve.............................TB-6, KI-6
Convulsion, stop by regulating qi flow and tendons LI-4, GB-34,

Damp-heat, clear in lower burner CV-3, SP-9
Damp-heat, eliminate in LV-GB LV-3, GB-34
Dampness, drain...SP-6, SP-9
Dampness, transform BL-20, SP-9
Deafness, sudden, empirical point for................................TB-16
Delivery, promote..BL-67
Diarrhea, infantile, empirical point for.............................M-UE-9 (*sifeng*) (bleed)
Discharge, check BL-30,BL-32, GB-36
Diuresis, promote to eliminate damp LI-6, SP-9, BL-28
Dizziness and vision, clear GV-20
Drain damp heat SP-9
Dysmenorrhea BL-32, SP-6, BL-60

Earth, supplement and replenish qi SP-3, ST-36
Epigastric fullness, relieve PC-6, CV-12,, ST-44
Exterior pathogens, resolve..LI-4, TB-5
Exterior, resolve and eliminate wind GV-16, GB-20, BL-12
Exterior, resolve by causing perspiration..............................LI-4, KI-7
Exterior, resolve to dispel wind pathogen LI-4, TB-5
Fetus,point for malposition ....BL-67†
Fever, high, reduce...Bleed hand *jing*-well
Fever, reduce...LI-11, GV-14
Fire, cool in heart and liver..PC-7, LV-2
Fire, liver, bring down GB-34, LV-2
Fire, liver-heart, drain PC-8, LV-2
Fluid, move CV-9, SP-9, BL-22
Food stagnation, relieve in stomach.................................LV-13, CV-10, ST-44
Foot yin channels, activate to strengthen genitourinary function................SP-6†
Furuncle, empirical point GV-10

Gastric and intestinal obstruction, relieve............................CV-10, ST-25
Gastrosplenic qi, supplement......................................BL-20†, BL-21†, ST-36†
Girdling vessel, stabilize...GB-26, GB-41
Governing vessel, remove obstruction and heat in GV-14, GV-13

Headache and nasal obstruction, relieve LU-7, LI-4, LI-20

Headache, frontal .... **LI-4, ST-8,** *yintang,* **GV-23, ST-44**

Headache, occipital SI-3, GB-20, BL-60

Headache, parietal **SI-3, GV-20, LV-3, BL-67**

Headache, temporal .... **TB-5, GB-8,** *taiyang,* **GB-41**

Heart fire (somatic as opposed to spirit-related), clear BL-14, PC-8

Heart fire (spirit-related), reduce HT-8, BL-15

Heart, calm, when yin depletion HT-7, KI-3

Heart, calm, when blood depletion HT-7, SP-6

Heart, clear and transform phlegm PC-5, ST-40

Heart, regulate BL-15, CV-14, PC-6

Heat, dissipate, clear mind PC-8, KI-1

Heat in blood, cool SP-10, LI-11, BL-40

Heat in channels, clear GV-14, LI-11, LI-4

Heat in governing channel, reduce GV-16, GV-14

Heat in lower yin channels, drain SP-6

Heat in pericardium channel, clear PC-8, PC-7

Heat in yang channels, clear GV-14

Heat in yangming channels, clear LI-11, ST-6, ST-44

Heat, cool and relieve stagnation in yangming channel LI-1, LI-11,

Heat, dispel in hand yangming channel LI-2, LI-11

Heat, dispel in triple burner channel TB-2, TB-5

Heat, disperse to relieve headache .... M-HN-9 (*taiyang*)

Heat, drain in upper body .... hand well-*jing* points

Heat, eliminate intense .... M-UE-1-5 (*shixuan*) (bleed)

Heat, extreme, manic cases .... Bleed well-*jing* points

Heat, reduce .... PC-3, BL-40 (bleed), *shixuan* (bleed)

Heat, resolve pathogenic LI-11

Heat, upper body, conduct downward KI-1

Hemoptysis, stop LU-6, BL-17

Hepatocystic damp-heat, dispel .... LV-3 toward KI-1, GB-34

Hypochondrium and breasts, relieve distention and pain in LV-14

Infantile diarrhea, empirical point for .... M-UE-9 (*sifeng*) (bleed)

Infantile malnutrition, empirical point for .... M-UE-9 (*sifeng*) (bleed)

Insomnia, generic treatment HT-7, SP-6

Intestinal dampness, clear SP-9, ST-43

Intestinal function, supplement LI-4, ST-25, ST-37

Intestinal heat, cool LI-11, ST-37, ST-44

Intestinal stagnation, relieve ST-25, ST-44

Intestines, regulate CV-6, ST-25

Intestines and stomach, clear damp heat from LI-11, ST-44, SP-9

Kidney essence, reinforce ....BL-23†
Kidney jing, supplement KI-3, BL-52
Kidney qi and essence, supplement ....BL-23†, CV-4†
Kidney qi, reinforce ....BL-23†, GV-4†, CV-6†
Kidney qi, strengthen to promote urination.......................CV-4†
Kidney qi, supplement ....BL-23†, GV-4†, KI-3
Kidney yang (mingmen), supplement ....GV-4†, BL-23†
Kidney yang, invigorate ....BL-23†, GV-4†, KI-3
Kidney yin, nourish KI-3
Kidney yin, strengthen to regulate menses KI-5
Kidney yin, supplement to nourish liver KI-3, SP-6
Kidney, strengthen...BL-23, KI-3
Kidney, supplement and nourish tendons..........................KI-6, LV-8
Kidney, supplement KI-3, BL-23

Lactation, empirical point...SI-1
Large intestine channel, reduce heat in LI-1, LI-11
Large intestine qi, supplement ....BL-25†, ST-37†
Large intestine, adjust function of.................................ST-25, ST-37
Large intestine, clear stagnation in................................ST-25, ST-37
Large intestine, regulate..ST-25, BL-25
Liver and gallbladder channels, regulate qi of LV-3, GB-41
Liver and gallbladder fire, dispel LV-2, GB-43
Liver and gallbladder, calm BL-18, BL-19
Liver yang, subdue BL-18, BL-23
Liver and kidney yin, supplement LV-3, KI-3
Liver and stomach fire, calm LV-2, LV-3, ST-44
Liver fire in head, clear..GB-12, GB-20
Liver fire, cool LV-2
Liver function, calm LV-3, LV-14
Liver gallbladder fire, reduce......................................LV-2, LV-3, GB-37
Liver qi stagnation, relieve LV-3, LV-14, GB-34
Liver qi, calm..LV-2, LV-3
Liver qi, clear stagnated..PC-6, LV-3
Liver qi, course stagnated LI-4, LV-3
Liver qi, harmonize..LV-3, LV-14
Liver qi, regulate..PC-6, LV-3
Liver wind, calm...LV-3
Liver yang, calm LV-2, BL-18, GB-20
Liver yin, nourish to reduce depletion fire LV-3, LV-8
Liver yin, soothe to promote patent flow.........................LV-3, LV-14
Liver, calm to promote patent qi flow LV-2
Liver, calm to relax diaphragm LV-3, LV-14
Liver, remove stagnation...BL-18, LV-1
Liver, soothe to relieve binding depression LV-3, BL-18
Lower burner, strengthen to promote intestinal function........CV-4, SP-6††
Lower burner, regulate and cool CV-3

Lower burner, reinforce circulation in ....SP-6†
Lower burner, supplement, reinforce essence.......................................CV-4†, BL-23†
Lower burner, warm to loosen bowels ....CV-6†, CV-8 (salt moxa)
Lung and stomach heat, reduce..LU-10, ST-44
Lung heat, cool LU-5
Lung heat, dissipate...LU-5, BL-13
Lung heat, drain...LU-11 (bleed)
Lung qi, activate, reinforce ....BL-13†, CV-17
Lung yin, activate...LU-7, KI-6
Lung, moisten to relieve cough LU-5
Lung-metal, strengthen by supplementing earth.................................LU-9, SP-3, ST-36

Marrow, nourish to relieve dizziness and tinnitus KI-3, GV-20
Mental clarity, restore..GV-26
Middle burner function, strengthen..SP-3, CV-12†, LV-13†
Middle burner qi, supplement..CV-12†, ST-36†
Middle burner, regulate..CV-12, SP-4
Middle burner, warm..CV-12†, CV-8 (salt moxa)

Mind, clear GV-26
Mind, resuscitate and clear GV-26, GV-20
Nasal obstruction, relieve ....M-HN-3 (*yintang*), LI-20, GV-26

Origin qi, supplement ....CV-4†

Palpitations and insomnia, calm...HT-7, SP-6
Pathogens in exterior, resolve LI-4, TB-5
Penetrating and conception vessels, regulate.....................................CV-7
Perspiration, promote by activating lung qi LU-7, LI-4
Phlegm in chest, resolve..PC-5, CV-22
Phlegm stagnation in middle burner, transform ST-40, SP-3
Promote qi circulation to relieve fullness LI-4, CV-6 ST-36
Pubic area, strengthen organs in ....LV-1†, LV-5†

Qi and blood, activate and harmonize LI-4, SP-6
Qi and blood, regulate to clear stagnation LI-4, SP-6
Qi and blood, supplement SP-6, ST-36
Qi in chest, regulate and restore milk flow.......................................PC-6, SI-1
Qi of *fu* organs, supplement..CV-12
Qi of yang channels, regulate..LI-4, ST-36
Qi of *zang* organs, supplement..LV-13
Qi, harmonize in shaoyang channels TB-2, GB-41
Qi in upper burner regulate CV-17
Qi, original, supplement ....CV-4†
Qi, precipitate to check hiccough SP-4, CV-22
Qi, recapture to reestablish yang ....CV-4, CV-6†, CV-8†(salt)
Qi, regulate in costal shaoyang channels...TB-6, GB-34

Qi, reinforce..CV-6†
Qi, source, warm and strengthen..CV-4†
Qi, stagnant in upper burner, disperse...................................CV-17
Qi, strengthen..CV-6
Qi, supplement and raise...CV-6†, GV-20†
Qi, supplement source qi ....CV-6†
Qi, supplement ....CV-6†, ST-36†
Qi and blood, promote circulation in yangming....................LI-4, ST-36
Qi and blood, promote in conception and penetrating vessels CV-6, KI-14

Rectal prolapse ....GV-20†, GV-1
Reinforce kidney qi...BL-23†, GV-4†
Respiratory function, regulate..BL-13, LU-1
Respiratory qi, regulate...CV-17
Resuscitation points (epilepsy)...GV-26, CV-15
Resuscitation, general..GV-26, PC-9

Spirit, calm HT-7
Spirit, calm and relieve depression..HT-7, LV-3
Spirit, fortify HT-7
Spirit, stabilize..SP-1
Spleen and kidney, regulate..BL-20†, BL-23†
Spleen and stomach, strengthen transporting function of ST-36
Spleen and stomach, strengthen...SP-3†, ST-36†
Spleen and stomach, supplement BL-20, ST-36, SP-6
Spleen and stomach, warm to dispel cold ....CV-6†, CV-12†, CV-13†
Spleen and kidney yang depletion, supplement ....CV-12†, BL-20†, BL-23†
Spleen qi, promote circulation..BL-20
Spleen qi, regulate SP-8
Spleen, regulate to drain damp-heat..SP-6, SP-9
Spleen, fortify to promote digestion LV-13
Spleen, strengthen to help harmonize stomach SP-4
Spleen, supplement to control blood ....ST-36, SP-1†, SP-6
Spleen and stomach yang, supplement.....................................BL-20†, BL-21†, CV-12†, LV-13†
Spleen and stomach, warm to dispel damp-cold ....CV-6†, CV-12†
Splenic yang, fortify...BL-20†
Splenogastric function, strengthen...SP-4†, ST-36†
Stomach and spleen, raise sunken qi of..................................GV-20†
Stomach channel heat, drain ST-44
Stomach qi counterflow, downbear..CV-17, CV-12, ST-36
Stomach qi, promote descent of..CV-12, ST-36

Stomach qi, supplement to reinforce spleen ST-36
Stomach, calm and check vomiting...PC-6, CV-12
Stomach, calm, and relieve stagnation ST-36, ST-44, ST-45

Thoracic and hypochondriac distress, relieve...............................TB-6, GB-34
Thoracic depression, relieve..PC-6, CV-17
Throat, sore TB-2, LU-10
Throat, cool..LU-10, LU-11 (bleed)
Trigeminal neuralgia, mandibular branch.....................................ST-44, ST-7,
                                                                                                           ST-6, CV-24
Trigeminal neuralgia, maxillary branch...LI-4, ST-2,
                                                                                                           ST-3. GV-26
Trigeminal neuralgia, ophthalmic branch......................................TB-5, GB-14
                                                                                                           taiyang, BL-2
Triple burner, clear TB-6,

Upper burner, regulate qi in...CV-17
Uterine bleeding, empirical points...LV-1, SP-1 (moxa only)
Uterine stasis, remove ST-29, BL-32
Uterus, lift ....M-CA-18 (*zigong*),
                                                                                                           ST-29†
Uterus, warm..CV-3†, CV-4†, ST-29†

Vital energy, strengthen...CV-4†, CV-6†
Vomiting, check and calm stomach PC-6, CV-12, ST-36
Vulvar, relieve itching LV-5

Water passages, supplement TB to promote circulation in.............TB-3, TB-4
Water passages, promote circulation in...BL-39
Wind and cold, eliminate ....LU-7, LI-4†
Wind, and heat, exogenous, expel LI-4, TB-5, GB-20
Wind in face (mouth awry) ST-4, ST-6
Wind in facial region, dispel..M-HN-9 (*taiyang*), LI-20
Wind in lower extremities...GB-30, GB-34,
                                                                                                           ST-36, ST-41
Wind in upper body GV-20, GV-16, BL-7
Wind in upper extremities LI-4, TB-5,
                                                                                                           LI-11, LI-15
Wind, dispel to relieve headache GB-20, GV-16, TB-5
Wind, liver, dispel LV-3
Wind, eliminate and secure exterior..GB-20, TB-5
Wind, eliminate, resolve the exterior GV-16, GB-20,
                                                                                                           BL-12, LU-7, LI-4
Wind, expel TB-5, GB-20
Wind, reduce and calm liver...GB-20, LV-3
Wind-heat, disperse TB-5, GB-20

Yang qi of spleen and kidney, invigorate...BL-20†, BL-23†
Yang qi, raise to support kidney ....GV-20†
Yang qi, raise ....CV-4†, GV-20†
Yang qi, reinforce and supplement kidney ....CV-4†, BL-23†, KI-7
Yang, invigorate ....SI-3, GV-4†, GV-14
Yang, raise in governing vessel..GV-26, GV-20†
Yang, raise ....GV-20†
Yang, revive and avert collapse CV-4, CV-6,
                                                                                                        CV-8 (salt)
Yang, supplement to dispel pathogen ....BL-12†, GV-14†
Yangming heat, drain..LI-4, LI-11, ST-44
Yin and blood, nourish KI-3, LV-3, SP-6
Yin channels, supplement lower ....SP-6†
Yin, regulate SP-6
Yin, supplement to reduce fire..KI-6, SP-6
Yin, supplement, activate descending function of lung LU-7, KI-6
Yin, supplement, to cool fire...KI-6

Part VII

Clinical Practice

19 Needling

19.1 "Clean Needle" Insertion Techniques

The necessity for maintaining clean insertion techniques cannot be overemphasized. The health of both patient and practitioner are at stake. By carefully following the recommendations first developed by the National Commission for the Certification of Acupuncturists in 1985, autogenic infection, hepatitis, and transmission of the AIDS virus can easily be prevented. Below are the seven basic steps necessary for clean needle insertion and treatment. For more detailed information, consult the manual, *Clean Needle Technique for Acupuncturists,* published by the NCCA.

Step 1:   **Washing up.** Wash hands thoroughly with soap and water or an alcohol-impregnated swab. Refrain from touching any contaminated area after washing.

Step 2:   **Establishing a clean field.** Lay out a clean field, such as uncontaminated paper towel, on a clean area, without contaminating it. Set out needles and other sterile equipment in the center of the clean field in such a way that they may be removed without contaminating the remaining needles and equipment on the field. Set your used-needle receptacle and wastebag outside, but close to, the clean field.

Step 3:   **Preparing the insertion site.** After locating the point, clean the site with an alcohol swab, rubbing in an outward spiral. Allow the alcohol to dry before inserting the needle. Avoid contaminating the site after cleaning it.

Step 4:   **Cleanly inserting the needle.** Wash hands *once again* with soap and water, or swab them thoroughly with an alcohol swab. Remove a needle from the clean field, maintaining sterility (i.e., without touching) of the needle shaft. If a insertion tube is used, put the needle into it handle first, keeping the tube clean. If the needle shaft is supported, hold it with sterile cotton or gauze.

        Note: For examination purposes, the needle will be inserted at least 1/4 inch, at both 90° and 45° angles.

Step 5:   **Cleanly manipulate the needle.** Whatever manipulation techniques you may use, whether rotating, thrusting and withdrawing, etc., do so *without touching the shaft or site with anything unsterile.*

        Note: For testing purposes, the needle is rotated clockwise one full turn.

Step 6.   **Cleanly withdraw the needle.** Withdraw the needle without touching the shaft or hole with your hands. If you wish to "close the hole," do so by applying pressure with clean cotton or gauze.

Step 7:   **Cleanly conclude the treatment.** Immediately dispose used needles in a container which should be clearly labeled "used needles" or "unsterile needles." Immediately dispose used cotton in a wastebag or similar receptacle, which should be lined with plastic. After disposing of all contaminated materials, once again, *wash your hands thoroughly.*

19.2 Supplementation and Draining Techniques

Many different methods for supplementing and draining acupuncture points have been developed over the centuries. Some have proven more clinically useful than others. Often, it is a question of the individual skill or particular approach of a practitioner which will determine what method will obtain the best results.

Supplementation and Drainage *(General Guidelines)*	
Indications for Supplementation	**Indications for Drainage**
Yin diseases (depleted, cold, chronic); support upright qi of body	Yang diseases (replete, febrile, acute); expel pathogen from body
For weak, depleted constitutional types	For strong, replete constitutional types
When skin feels relaxed and flaccid upon palpation	When skin feels tight, painful, or nodular upon palpation

Below are fifteen techniques that have proven most useful in clinical practice. They represent modification of four basic aspects of needling:

> *The needle itself;*
>
> *The actual insertion of the needle through the skin;*
>
> *The manipulation of the needle after insertion; and*
>
> *The acupoint itself*

Learning them thoroughly and keeping them in mind every time you insert a needle will help focus your mind upon the treatment and cannot but have a beneficial effect.

15 Supplementing—Draining Needle Skills			
Aspect of Needling	**Parameter Controlled**	**To Supplement**	**To Drain**
The Needle	**Temp.**	Heat prior to insertion	Do not heat
	Gauge	Use thinner gauge	Use thicker gauge
The Insertion	**Speed**	Insert slowly and remove quickly	Insert quickly and remove slowly
	Depth	Insert shallowly	Insert more deeply
	Direction	Insert needle in direction of channel flow	Insert needle against channel flow
	Sensation	Do not cause sensation when needling	Elicit sensation when needling
	Vibration	Insert needle calmly and smoothly	Vibrate needle during insertion and removal
	Timing	Insert on exhalation, remove on inhalation	Insert on inhalation, remove on exhalation
The Manipulation	**Twirling**	Twirl clockwise	Twirl counterclockwise
	Retention	Leave the needle for more time	Leave the needle for less time
	Lifting & Thrusting	Thrust with force, lift gently	Lift with force, press gently
The Acupoint	**Massage**	Lightly rub the point before insertion	Insert without rubbing
	Pressure	Press or "close" the point after removal	Spread skin to "open" the point after removal
	Pinching	Pinch with the nails before insertion	Insert without pinching
	Point Selection	Needle the "mother" point (and channel)	Needle the "child" point (and channel)

19.3 Needle Contraindications

Needle Contraindications	
Point	**Comment**
GV-24	This point is now commonly needled .2-.3″
GV-17	Modern sources needle to .3″
BL-9	Currently needled .3″
BL-8	Currently needled .3-.5″
GB-18	Currently needled .3-.5″
TB-19	Currently needled .1″
TB-20	Currently needled .1″
ST-1	Currently needled .2-.3″; it can create a black eye - rarely used
GV-11	Some modern sources allow .5-1.0 inch insertion here
GV-10	See GV-11
CV-17	Now needled to a depth of .3-.5″
LI-13	Sight of the radial collateral artery and vein
HT-2	Currently needled .3-.5″
CV-8	At the navel, forbidden to needle - salt moxa only
KI-11	Currently needled .5-.8″
ST-30	This is the site of a major artery; currently needled .3-.5″
SP-11	Currently needled .3-.5″; it is the site of a major vein and artery
BL-56	Some modern sources needle this point 1.0-1.5″
CV-9	Currently needled .5-1.0″. Should not be needled to treat water swelling (employ moxibustion)

(Continued)

Needle Contraindications *(Continued)*	
Point	**Comment**
CV-1	Currently needled .5-.8″
ST-17	The nipple, forbidden to needle or apply direct moxa: use indirect moxa only
TB-8	Some modern sources needle this point .5-1.0″
LV-12	Site of femoral artery

Contraindications in Pregnancy

LI-4, SP-6, GB-21, and any abdominal points at any time during pregnancy; *8 liao (BL-31-34)* during the first and second trimesters

20 Moxibustion

20.1 Direct moxibustion

20.1.1 Scarring moxibustion

Direct scarring moxibustion is used to treat serious depletion cold or cold-damp diseases. Moxa cones varying in size from a millet seed to a small bean are placed directly on an acupoint and completely burned. This process is repeated several times, after which the skin is cleaned and dressed. Within a few days, a blister will form that will take about a month to heal. Because of its potential for scarring, this method is rarely used in the West. However, it should be acknowledged that this is a very potent and efficacious form of treatment.

20.1.2 Non-scarring moxibustion

Non-scarring moxibustion is similar to scarring moxibustion, except that the burning cones are extinguished with the fingers just before (or just as) they burn the skin, or are quickly removed with tweezers just before the skin is burned. In addition, smaller cones are used. This method is used for milder depletion cold patterns.

20.2 Indirect moxibustion

Indirect Moxibustion		
Technique	**Number of Cones Used**	**Application**
On salt (in umbilicus)	Up to 100 cones	Cold damage yin patterns, cholera, windstrike desertion patterns
On garlic (0.2" thick)	4-5 cones per slice, repeated 5 to 7 times per treatment	Depletion taxation (tuberculosis), toxicity from sores, scrofulous swellings, abdominal accumulation masses (may cause blistering)
On ginger (0.2" thick)	4-5 cones per slice, repeated 5 to 7 times per treatment	Middle burner depletion, abdominal fullness, stomach pain, *shan* pain, diarrhea, vomiting, wind-cold *bi* pain, wind-cold exterior patterns, yang depletion diseases
On aconite powder (fu zi)	Burn moxa cones on a small amount of powdered aconite placed on the point	Yang depletion diseases, prolonged lesions and boils

Moxa poles

Moxa poles are held about one inch above the acupoint and either moved in a circular motion or in an up-and-down, pecking motion until the patient feels a sensation of warmth. Several points are heated in succession, until the patient feels heat immediately upon bringing the pole near the point.

Moxa poles provide mild supplementation and are especially useful in treating wind-damp *bi* and similar patterns.

21 Cupping and Bloodletting

21.1 Cupping

Cupping is a therapeutic method whereby suction is applied to the skin surface by attaching a small jar of glass, porcelain, or bamboo in which a vacuum is created, either by introducing heat into the jar, or by a suction device attached to the top of the jar. It is often used for problems of wind, damp, numbness, or pain. It may be used by itself, or in conjunction with needles, moxa, or massage.

Cupping is indicated in a variety of conditions, though there are six general areas in which cupping is most commonly applied:

Cupping: Clinical Applications	
General Disorder	**Specific Application**
Respiratory	Cough, asthma, whooping cough
Musculo-Skeletal	Any tendon or bone pain (such as backache, sore legs, shoulder pain, etc.); sprains and twisted joints
Generalized Aches and Pains	Rheumatic or arthritic pain
Gastrointestinal Disorders	Stomachache, nausea
Menstrual	Menstrual problems or discharge
Headcolds and Flu	Headache, vertigo, swollen eyes from cold or flu

There are three varieties of cupping: dry cupping, wet cupping, and sliding cupping. Dry cupping involves placing the suction cups directly over the skin. Wet cupping involves first gently tapping the skin with a plum-blossom or seven-star needle to slightly perforate the skin, and then applying suction cups. Sliding cupping involves first applying an ointment (such as vaseline) over the area to be cupped, and then, when suction has been achieved, sliding the cups over the affected area.

21.1.1 Typical Cupping Treatments

Typical Cupping Treatments	
Disorder	**Cupping Treatment**
Asthma	BL-11, BL-13, GV-12, CV-12, CV-6
Cramps in the calf	BL-57, BL-40, SP-6
Dysentery	ST-25 (left), CV-12
German measles	GV-14, GV-4, LI-11, BL-40
Headache	GV-14, M-HN-9 (*taiyang*)
Headcold	M-HN-9 (*taiyang*), M-HN-3 (*yintang*), LI-4
Leukorrhea	CV-4, CV-6, SP-6
Malarial disease, tidal fevers	GV-14, GV-13
Menstrual pain	CV-6, CV-3, CV-4, ST-25, BL-23
Nausea or diarrhea	ST-25, CV-6, CV-4, SP-6, BL-20
Sprained joints or other injuries	Local points
Upper back pain	GV-14, GV-12, BL-11, BL-13
Whooping cough	GV-12

(Compiled from *Zhenjiu Jingwei* and *Linchuang Quxue Tujie*. For further examples of cupping treatments see therapy sections of *ECA* and *CAM*.)

21.1.2 Eight general precautions and contraindications for cupping

Cupping should not be used:

> —*Over the heart;*
>
> —*On the breast or abdomen during pregnancy;*
>
> —*In any area of skin-disease, edema, tumors, swollen lymph nodes, or pox eruptions;*
>
> —*Where the skin is dry and parched, or has lost all elasticity;*
>
> —*In cases of sudden fainting, coma, or convulsions;*
>
> —*In cases of violent cramps of the limbs;*
>
> —*Over large blood vessels, or on people with hemorrhagic tendency;*
>
> —*Where the marks from previous cupping have not yet completely disappeared.*

Some sensitive patients may become dizzy, nauseated, chilled, or faint; they may break out in a cold sweat or their complexion may go ashen or white. This is equivalent to "needle-shock" and should be handled in the same manner.

21.2 Bloodletting

Bloodletting is a method used to drain heat, quicken blood and qi, and relieve local congestion to reduce stagnation and swelling. Traditionally, the three-cornered needle was used, but a presterilized, disposable lancet will give the same results. The acupoint is first pressed to restrict blood flow, then quickly pricked to a depth of about 0.1″, after which a few drops of blood are squeezed out. If the blood appears dark or clotted, keep squeezing until red, clean blood appears.

Acupuncture Points Suitable for Bloodletting	
Disease	**Points for Bloodletting**
Wind strike	BL-40, LI-4, GB-21
Cholera	BL-40, LU-5, LI-11
Spasm of the gastrocnemius	SP-1
Cough (with phlegm)	LI-11, LU-5
Headache	ST-8, GV-20
Stomach (epigastric) pain	BL-38
Abdominal pain	LV-1
Ingesta damage	GV-20
Jaundice	SP-1, BL-20, BL-21
Spinal pain	BL-38
Hypochondriac pain	BL-18
Shan qi	BL-23
Mouth and tongue ulcers	HT-7
Swelling of mouth, tongue, or pharynx	LI-11
Toothache	LI-4
Wind, swelling and pain (in eyes)	ST-8
All eye diseases	BL-18, ST-8, LU-11, GV-20
Sore throat	LU-11
Drinker's nose	LU-7, LI-4
Strangury diseases	SP-6, BL-40
Foot qi	BL-57
Shoulder pain	BL-13
Itching over the entire body	LI-4, GV-20
Breast swelling and pain (in women)	BL-38
Menstrual clots	BL-40
Infantile *gan* disease	BL-18, BL-17, BL-21, GV-12, M-BW-24 and M-UE-9
Cinnabar toxicity (erysipelas)	BL-40, BL-17

Appendix

The Overview Tables

General Yin-Yang Relationships	
Phenomena	Space, Time, Season, Gender, Temperature, Weight, Brightness, Motion
Anatomy and Physiology	Parts of the body Tissues and Organs Activity and Function
Pathology	Disorders, Pulses
Imbalances	Signs of Yang Repletion Signs of Yin Repletion

Qi, Blood, Fluids, Essence		
Qi	*Five Functions of Qi*	Activation, Warming, Defense, Transformation, Containment
	Fifteen Types of Qi	Prenatal, Postnatal, Cosmic, Grain, True, Correct, Evil, Organ, Channel, Construction, Defense, Ancestral, Center, Clear, Turbid
	Four Disorders of Qi	Qi Depletion, Qi Stagnation, Qi Counterflow, Qi Fall
Blood	*Three Aspects of Blood*	Governed by the Heart Stored by the Liver Managed by the Spleen
	Three Disorders of Blood	Blood Depletion, Blood Stasis, Blood Heat
Fluid	*Two Types of Fluid*	Liquid, Humor
	Four Disorders of Fluid	Damage to Liquid, Humor Desertion, Water Swelling, Phlegm-Rhuem (*tan-yin*)
Essence	*Four Types of Essence*	Congenital, Acquired, Reproductive, Essential

The Organs

Zang Organs	Heart, Lung, Spleen, Liver, Kidney, Heart Governor ("Pericardium")
Fu Organs	Small Intestine, Large Intestine, Stomach, Gallbladder, Bladder, Triple Burner
Curious Organs	Brain, Marrow, Bone, Blood Vessels, Uterus, and Gallbladder (simultaneously considered a *fu* organ)
Zang-Fu Pairs	Heart - Small Intestine Lung - Large Intestine Spleen - Stomach Liver - Gallbladder Kidney - Bladder Heart Governor - Triple Burner

Channels and Vessels

The Major Channels	**12** Regular Channels **8** Irregular Vessels
The Connecting Vessels	**15** Major Connecting Vessels (*luo mai*) **Numerous** Reticular Connecting Vessels (*sun luo*)
Channel Sinews and Channel Divergences	**12** Channel Sinews (*Tendino-muscular meridians*) **12** Channel Divergences

The Major Channels

The Twelve Regular Channels	Each has an organ to which it **homes** Each has an organ with which it **connects** Each is linked with another in an **interior-exterior pair** Each yin channel **communicates** with another yin channel, and each yang channel with another yang channel Each may be distinguished by its relative proportions of qi and blood
The Eight Irregular Vessels	They are employed in **coupled** pairs Each is accessed via a **master point**

17 Important Point Types and Categories	
Point Category	**Summary**
Transporting-*shu* Points	**5** points per channel: also called "Antique;" important in five-phase applications.
Mother-Child Points	**1** Mother (supplementing) and **1** Child (draining) point for each channel.
Back Transporting-*shu* Points	**12** points, all on the back along the spine, each relating to a specific organ; also called "Associated" or "Assent" points.
Front Alarm-*mu* Points	**12** points, all on the torso, each relating to a specific organ; also called "Herald" points.
Source-*yuan* Points	**12** points, one per channel, each in direct communication with the channel's associated organ.
Connecting-*luo* Points	**15** points, one per each major channel (each the point of departure for the channel's connecting vessel) and one each for the Conception and Governing vessels, plus the "Great *luo* Point," SP-21.
Meeting-*hui* Points	**8** points, each with a therapeutic effect on a specific tissue group, region, or function.
Cleft-*xi* Points	**16** points, used in acute, painful or stubborn situations.
Master-*jiaohui* Points	**8** points, also called "confluent points," one for each of the eight irregular vessels; usually paired when used in clinical practice.
Lower Uniting-*he* Points	**6** points, each having a direct and powerful effect on an associated *fu* organ.

(Continued)

17 Important Point Types and Categories
(Continued)

Point Category	Summary
General Connecting-*luo* Points	**5** points (2 yang, 3 yin), affecting the Irregular Vessels, used to balance yin and yang; particularly effective before treatment.
Group Connecting-*luo* Points	**4** points, used to unite all the yin channels on the upper limbs, to unite all the yang channels on the upper limbs, and, similarly, to unite all the yin and yang channels on the lower limbs.
Command Points	**4** points, one each with a powerful effect on the abdomen, back, head, and face/mouth.
The Four Seas	**2** points each for the Seas of Nourishment and Marrow, **3** points each for the Seas of Qi and Blood.
Windows of the Sky Points	**5** points, each with a specific symptomatology relating to the inability of the yang qi to rise to the head.
Entry and Exit Points	**12** points, each connecting one channel to the next in the "Chinese clock" cycle (superficial circulation of qi) via a secondary vessel.
Intersection Points	Points where several channels cross. These are points where qi and blood easily become bound and congested; needling these points will have a beneficial effect on several channels at once (see table at section **8.15**).

Causes of Illness

Six Exogenous Causes	Wind, Cold, Fire, Damp, Summerheat, Dryness
Seven Endogenous Causes	Joy, Anger, Anxiety, Preoccupation Support, Fear, Fright
Five Independent Causes	Dietary Irregularity, Excessive Sexual Activity, Taxation Fatigue, Trauma, Parasites
Two Additional Causes	Phlegm, Static Blood

Patterns of Illness	
Pattern Category	**Patterns**
Eight Parameter Patterns	Exterior and Interior Hot and Cold Repletion and Depletion Yang and Yin
Qi-Blood Patterns	Qi Depletion Patterns Qi Stagnation Patterns Qi Fall Patterns Qi Counterflow Patterns Blood Depletion Patterns Blood Stasis Patterns Blood Heat Patterns
Zang-fu Patterns	Heart (6), Lung (4), Spleen (3), Stomach/Spleen (4), Liver (10), Kidney (11) Stomach (3), Small Intestine (3), Large Intestine (2), Gallbladder (2), Bladder (2). *Numbers in parenthesis indicate number of patterns presented*
Pathogen Patterns	Wind, Cold, Heat and Fire, Summerheat, Damp, Dry, Digestate Accumulation, Phlegm.
Exogenous Heat Patterns	*Six-Channel Patterns:* Taiyang, Shaoyang, Yangming, Taiyin, Shaoyin, Jueyin
	Four-Aspect Patterns Defense (*wei*), Qi, Construction (*ying*), Blood
	Triple Burner Patterns Upper Burner (Lung and Pericardium) Middle Burner (Stomach and Spleen) Lower Burner (Liver and Kidney)
	Pericardiac Patterns Inward Fall of Pathogens to the Pericardium Clouding of the Pericardium by Phlegm Turbidity Stomach Heat Sweltering the Pericardium

Zang-Fu Patterns	
Organ	**Potential Disorders**
Heart	Heart Qi Depletion Heart Yang Depletion Heart Blood Depletion Heart Yin Depletion Upflaming of Heart Fire Cardiac *Bi*
Lung	Non-Diffusion of Lung Qi Impaired Depurative Downbearing of Lung Qi Lung Qi Depletion Lung Yin Depletion
Spleen	Spleen Qi Depletion Devitalization of Splenic Yang Center Qi Fall
Stomach/Spleen	Blood Management Failure Gastric Qi Depletion Cold Insufficiency of Stomach Yin
Liver	General Binding Depression of Liver Qi Invasion of the Stomach by Liver Qi Hepatosplenic Disharmony Plumstone Globus Struma Disorders of the Governing and Penetrating Vessels Upflaming of Liver Fire Ascendant Hyperactivity of Liver Yang Liver Wind Liver Blood Depletion

(Continued)

Zang-Fu Patterns *(Continued)*	
Organ	**Potential Disorder**
Kidney	Kidney Yin Depletion Cardiorenal Yin Depletion Hepatorenal Yin Depletion Pulmorenal Yin Depletion Kidney Yang Depletion Splenorenal Yang Depletion Qi-Absorption Failure Cardiorenal Yang Debilitation Yang Depletion Water Flood Insufficiency of Kidney Essence Insecurity of Kidney Qi
Stomach	Stomach Heat Stomach Yin Insufficiency Stomach Cold Stomach Qi Depletion Epigastric Food Stagnation
Small Intestine	Depletion Cold of the Small Intestine Repletion Heat of the Small Intestine Small Intestine Qi Pain
Large Intestine	Large Intestine Repletion Heat Large Intestine Damp Heat Large Intestine Fluid Depletion Intestinal Depletion Efflux Desertion Large Intestine Depletion Cold
Gallbladder	Gallbladder Repletion Gallbladder Depletion
Bladder	Bladder Damp Heat Bladder Depletion Cold

Pathogen Patterns	
Pathogen	**Potential Illness Pattern**
Wind	Contraction of Exogenous Wind Invasion of the Channels by the Wind Pathogen Wind Cold Damp *Bi*
Cold	Contraction of the Cold Pathogen Cold *Bi* Cold Pain Cold Diarrhea Cold *Shan*
Heat and Fire	Repletion Heat Depletion Heat
Summerheat	Summerheat Heat Summerheat Damp
Damp	Damp Obstruction Damp-Heat Lodged in the Qi Aspect (in T.B.) Splenogastric Damp Obstruction Brewing Hepatocystic Damp-Heat Downpour of Damp-Heat into the Large Intestine Downpour of Damp-Heat into the Bladder
Dryness	Contraction of Exogenous Dryness Damage to Liquid Damage to Yin Blood Dryness
Phlegm	Damp Phlegm Cold Phlegm Heat Phlegm Wind-Phlegm Phlegm Confounding the Cardiac Portals Phlegm Lodging in the Channels or Limbs Phlegm Lodging in the Chest and Hypochondrium
Digestate Accumulation	Ingesta Damage Gastrointestinal Accumulation Splenic Depletion with Ingesta Damage Complication

Exogenous Heat Patterns	
Six-Channel Patterns	Taiyang, Shaoyang, Yangming, Taiyin, Shaoyin, Jueyin
Four-Aspect Patterns	Defense (*wei*), Qi, Construction (*ying*), Blood
Triple Burner Patterns	Upper Burner (Lung and Pericardium) Middle Burner (Stomach and Spleen) Lower Burner (Liver and Kidney)
Pericardiac Patterns	Inward Fall of Pathogens to the Pericardium Clouding of the Pericardium by Phlegm Turbidity Stomach Heat Sweltering the Pericardium

Six Channel Patterns		
`Pattern	Pathomechanism	Manifestations
Taiyang	Assailment of the exterior by wind cold	Exterior Repletion Exterior Depletion
Yangming	Gastrointestinal repletion heat	Channel Pattern Bowel Pattern
Shaoyang	Pathogen at midstage between exterior and interior	Exterior Pattern Interior Pattern
Taiyin	Gastrointestinal depletion cold	Like *yangming* bowel pattern but with signs of depletion
Shaoyin	Cardiorenal debilitation	Depletion Cold Depletion Heat
Jueyin	Interior depletion and cold/heat complex	Upper body heat with lower body cold

Four Aspect Patterns		
Pattern	**Pathomechanism**	**Differentiation**
Defense	Pathogen in the defensive exterior	Wind Thermia Damp Thermia
Qi	Exuberant heat in the qi aspect	First Stage Qi Aspect Heat Exuberant Pulmogastric Heat Great Heat in the Qi Aspect Gastrointestinal Heat Bind Heat Lodging in the Triple Burner Brewing Damp-Heat Steaming the Intestines and Stomach
Construction	Inward fall of pathogenic heat to the construction aspect	Inward Fall of Thermia Heat or Wind Thermia Inward Fall of Damp Thermia
Blood	Penetration of pathogenic heat to the blood aspect, causing depletion or frenetic blood movement	Repletion Heat at the Blood Aspect Depletion Heat at the Blood Aspect

Methods of Diagnosis	
Observation	Spirit, Complexion, Excretions, Appearance, Tongue,
Audio-Olfaction	Listening, Smelling
Enquiry	Chills and Fever; Perspiration; Thirst, Appetite, Taste; Defecation and Urination; Pain; Hearing and Vision; Sleep; Menstruation Childbirth; History; Emotions, Lifestyle, Home and Work Environment
Palpation	Pulse Examination, Palpation of Channels and Points, Abdominal Palpation

Bibliography

English References

Beijing College of Traditional Chinese Medicine, et al. *Essentials of Chinese Acupuncture.* Beijing: Foreign Languages Press, 1980.

_____. *Chinese Acupuncture and Moxibustion.* Beijing: Foreign Languages Press, 1988.

Hoc Ku Huynh, trans. *Pulse Diagnosis* (translation of Li Shizhen's *Binhu Moxue,* 1564). Brookline, MA.: Paradigm Publications, 1985.

Mann, Felix. *Acupuncture, the Ancient Chinese Art of Healing.* Second edition. London: William Heinemann Medical Books Ltd., 1971

Matsumoto, Kiiko and Steven Birch. *Extraordinary Vessels.* Brookline, MA: Paradigm Publications, 1986.

_____.*Hara Diagnosis: Reflections on the Sea.* Brookline, MA: Paradigm Publications, 1988.

O'Connor, J. and Dan Bensky, trans. *Acupuncture, a Comprehensive Text.* Chicago: Eastland Press, 1981.

Porkert, Manfred. *Theoretical Foundations of Chinese Medicine.* M.I.T. East Asian Sciences Series, Vol. 3. Cambridge, MA: M.I.T. Press, 1974.

Unschuld, Paul U., trans. *Nan-Ching: the Classic of Difficult Issues.* Berkeley, Los Angeles, London: University of California Press, 1986.

Wiseman, Nigel et al. *Fundamentals of Chinese Acupuncture.* Brookline, MA: Paradigm Publications, 1988.

_____. *Fundamentals of Chinese Medicine.* Brookline, MA: Paradigm Publications, 1987.

Chinese References

Beijing Institute of Traditional Chinese Medicine, et al. *Zhongguo Zhenjiuxue Gaiyao* (Essentials of Chinese Acupuncture). Beijing: People's Health Press, 1980.

Ch'uang Yu-min. *Zhenjiu Linchuang Shouci* (Acumoxa Clinical Handbook). Taipei: Privately published, 1974.

Nanjing Institute of Traditional Chinese Medicine. *Zhongyixue Gailun* (Introduction to Chinese Medicine). Beijing: People's Health Press, 1959.

Shanghai Institute of Traditional Chinese Medicine. *Zhongyixue Jichu* (Fundamentals of Chinese Medicine). Beijing: Peoples Health Press, 1975

_____. *Zhenjiuxue* (Acumoxatherapy). Beijing: People's Health Press, 1974.

Yang Wei-chieh, ed. *Huangdi Neijing Yijie* (Annotated Yellow Emperor's Inner Canon). Taipei: Lien Kuo Publishing House, 1984.

_____. *Zhenjiu Wushuxue Yingyung* (Utilizing the Five Transport Acupoints). Taipei: Le Ch'un Publishing Co., 1981.

Zhenjiu Dacheng Jiaoshi (Corrected and Explained 'Great Compendium of Acumoxa'). No editors listed. Taipei: Ch'i Yeh Publishing, 1987.

General Index